Healthcare Reform in America

Books in the **Contemporary World Issues** series address vital issues in today's society such as genetic engineering, pollution, and biodiversity. Written by professional writers, scholars, and nonacademic experts, these books are authoritative, clearly written, up-to-date, and objective. They provide a good starting point for research by high school and college students, scholars, and general readers as well as by legislators, businesspeople, activists, and others.

Each book, carefully organized and easy to use, contains an overview of the subject, a detailed chronology, biographical sketches, facts and data and/or documents and other primary source material, a forum of authoritative perspective essays, annotated lists of print and nonprint resources, and an index.

Readers of books in the Contemporary World Issues series will find the information they need to have a better understanding of the social, political, environmental, and economic issues facing the world today.

Healthcare Reform in America

A REFERENCE HANDBOOK

Second Edition

Jennie Jacobs Kronenfeld and
Michael Kronenfeld

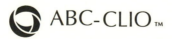

An Imprint of ABC-CLIO, LLC
Santa Barbara, California • Denver, Colorado

Library of Congress Cataloging-in-Publication Data

Kronenfeld, Jennie J., author.

  Healthcare reform in America : a reference handbook / Jennie Jacobs Kronenfeld and Michael Kronenfeld. — Second edition.

    p. ; cm. — (Contemporary world issues)

  Includes bibliographical references and index.

  ISBN 978–1–61069–965–5 (hard copy : alk. paper) — ISBN 978–1–61069–966–2 (eISBN) I. Kronenfeld, Michael R., author. II. Title. III. Series: Contemporary world issues. [DNLM: 1. Health Care Reform—United States. 2. Federal Government—United States. 3. Quality of Health Care—economics—United States. WA 540 AA1]

RA395.A3

362.1'04250973—dc23   2014045767

ISBN: 978–1–61069–965–5
EISBN: 978–1–61069–966–2

19 18 17 16 15   2 3 4 5

This book is also available on the World Wide Web as an eBook.
Visit www.abc-clio.com for details.

ABC-CLIO, LLC
130 Cremona Drive, P.O. Box 1911
Santa Barbara, California 93116-1911

This book is printed on acid-free paper ∞

Manufactured in the United States of America

Depending on how one views the Patient Protection and Affordable Care Act (PPACA, more commonly referred to as ACA), passed in 2010 during the first term of the presidency of Barack Obama, the United States has either passed major health reform legislation, major health insurance reform, or legislation that may destroy many of the positive changes to healthcare in the United States in the past 50 years. The ACA is the most important change in the healthcare system in the United States since passage of Medicare and Medicaid in 1965. It is attempting to greatly improve access to care, provide a more consistent quality of care for all Americans, and address cost issues. The limited reforms that occurred in the 1990s (some control of managed care; the CHIP program) and the addition of drug coverage to the Medicare program addressed these issues in a more piecemeal fashion. Due to the ACA, some important concerns such exceeding the amount of coverage after developing a major health problem and lack of coverage for preexisting conditions have been addressed.

This handbook reviews both successful and failed attempts at healthcare reform in the past century, identifying the economic, social, and political issues that both pushed for the creation of a national system and prevented it from being completely implemented. Most experts agree that some very important issues remain. While there have been some efforts at cost control and quality improvement, there will continue to be concerns that require additional changes in administration, technology, and training. Issues of long-term healthcare needs for older adults, people with disabilities, and people with chronic mental illness will also need to be addressed.

This handbook on healthcare reform presents issues and questions relevant to the full range of social science disciplines in high school and college-level courses. By showing the interplay and significance of these issues as they focus on the healthcare system, the reader should be able to see the importance and interplay of the work of the different disciplines on the topic.

This book is very different than it would have been if it had been written 20 years ago, before the emergence of the Internet as an increasingly important platform for the presentation of information, analysis, and advocacy on the relevant (and sometimes not so relevant) issues of our time. Before the Web, access to information and viewpoints on a topic were both limited and often not timely. While many issue advocacy groups existed before the Internet, finding out about them was both difficult and time consuming. Government data were available at many public and academic libraries but were hard to find and access. Periodical indexes were available at libraries, but tracking down the articles identified was much more difficult and time consuming. While many of the issues relating to the healthcare sector and the delivery of healthcare in the United States have not greatly changed in this time period, the ability to access information on the topic has grown almost exponentially.

The ability to access large volumes of information has not made the task of understanding the issues any easier for someone just beginning to explore and understand them. It is very easy to become overwhelmed both with the volume of information and with the worthiness of the information presented by competing and contradictory advocacy groups. The first two chapters of the book introduce the reader to the basic issues and give the context needed to further explore the issues discussed in some of the later chapters. The third and fourth chapters provide beginning researchers perspectives on how different experts see the promises and challenges arising from the passage of the ACA, as well as introduce them to some of the key players in the recent efforts of reforming our healthcare system. Chapters 5 and 6 provide basic data on the healthcare system and identify sources for additional research. Finally, the Glossary and Chronology provide ready reference to assist the reader in understanding the terminology of the healthcare system and its reform as well as the over 200-year history of its development.

Viewing and understanding the U.S. healthcare system is similar to the issue of different people viewing the proverbial elephant. It is a large and complicated animal that looks and feels very different depending on the perspective of the viewer and which aspect of the system is being viewed. In this handbook, the authors have attempted to give the new researcher the background and the resources to view and understand the parts of the system within the context of the whole system, which takes up almost 20 percent of the U.S. economy, directly impacting the life and health of all of Americans.

Healthcare Reform in America

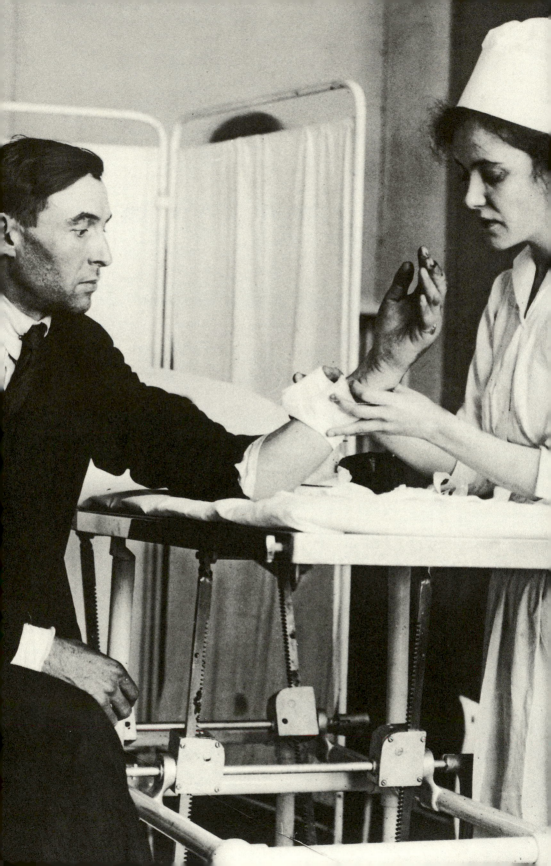

Healthcare reform, or modification of the U.S. healthcare system so that affordable, high-quality healthcare services are available to everyone, is a public policy issue that has, off and on, been discussed in the United States since World War II. How *much* discussion varies with changes in who the leading politicians are and how much healthcare issues are viewed as issues of high public concern. The past decade has been one of those periods of heightened interest in healthcare reform issues in the United States, culminating with the passage of the Affordable Care Act in 2010.

Introduction

In recent decades, the prominence of the topic of healthcare reform has varied. It was a central issue in the first term of the Clinton administration but moved to a position of lower concern by Clinton's second term. During the administration of George W. Bush, the events of September 11, 2001, led to a greater focus on international concerns and terrorism, and the prominence of healthcare issues became fairly low. With the election of Barack Obama as president in 2008, the issue of healthcare reform again became one of the major issues in the

---

A Public Health Service nurse treats a patient in the early 1900s. (Library of Congress)

political discourse. The Affordable Care Act was passed only after major debates and controversies, which have continued to be a major issue politically throughout the first two years of Obama's second term. The specifics of the debates over passage of this legislation, the legislation itself, and the continuing issues with its initial implementation are covered in more detail in Chapter 2 of this book. Much of the rest of this chapter will cover background and history prior to Obama's reform efforts.

Compared to almost all other industrialized countries in the world today, the United States has not resolved some very basic issues about the role of the government in the provision of care and in ensuring that all citizens are able to receive care of good quality when they need it. In most of the world's industrialized countries, the government has been part of a process that guarantees access to many, if not most, healthcare services to all citizens. Not all countries arrive at the same solution for guaranteeing access to all. Some create a major national healthcare system (e.g., Great Britain); others use more of a health insurance–based system. These can vary widely. In Canada, there is a single-payer national health insurance system that, over the years, some have believed could be a model for how to reform U.S. healthcare. The system in Canada varies from one province to another (provinces are more or less the equivalent of U.S. states), and most physicians are still paid by health insurance, rather than on a yearly or per patient salary. In Germany, nongovernmental insurance providers form the basis of the system, but there are various mechanisms in place to ensure that all Germans are covered for most services. Many argue that the United States does not really have a clear healthcare system; instead, a confusing variety of public and private healthcare insurers and providers function in different, and often competing, ways. Thus, while most countries have mechanisms in place to ensure at least basic access to healthcare to all, and to maintain quality while keeping overall costs reasonable, this is not true of the United States.

For almost 50 years, cost, quality, and access have been the three key watchwords for scholars in many of the different disciplines that study healthcare and the delivery of healthcare services. The name given to these types of studies and studies related to many aspects of the healthcare system is health services research. This name started to be used about 30 years ago to describe research related to the use of, organization and delivery of, financing of, and outcomes of health services such as quality of care and health status changes. Over the last 15 years, it has become the most widely accepted term to describe interdisciplinary research on health and healthcare services. Disciplines that are often part of health services research include sociology, economics, political science, management sciences, epidemiology, and more applied fields such as public health, health services administration, health education, and policy sciences.

The importance of these three concepts (cost, quality, and access) should not be surprising, and apply to many kinds of services that a person might receive, not just healthcare. For any service (or product), one thing of importance is how much does it cost? For an individual about to visit a physician (or a store), the simple question is what must I pay? The more complicated question is whether the price is fair, reasonable, and appropriate. When this question is applied beyond the individual to a large group or the nation as a whole, we begin to ask questions such as what are the total dollars being spent, how do these dollars relate to other kinds of services, and how do they relate to how much people in other places pay for these kinds of services?

A related question is can I get the service or product? This is the concept of access. Access has at least two components, and one component is simply the availability of the service. Are there physicians or hospitals around? Are the physicians taking new patients? Do the hospitals have empty beds? In healthcare, this question is often termed geographical access and is linked to specific places. While the answers to policy questions about geographical access can be complex, the more complex side of access is financial access, or do I have the money to pay for care? Increasingly in the United States, the answer to this question relates less to the amount of money any individual has in his or her wallet or bank account, and more to whether the person (and the person's family) has health insurance. The most important factor in having health insurance in the United States before the Obama reforms has been having a good job with benefits. In addition, certain categories of people, such as older adults, many of the poor, and increasingly the children of the near poor now have access to government-sponsored health insurance. Thus, access for an individual is partially linked to cost of care and also to specific aspects of that person's situation in society. It is easy to see how access issues quickly become one major group of issues in healthcare reform.

Moving beyond the individual to society as a whole, cost of care is linked to access, and at a broader policy level, this is particularly true. If a governmental unit, such as a state, is willing or able to spend a certain amount on healthcare for the poor and those without insurance, the state can provide more access to care to greater numbers of people if the average cost of care per person is $500 versus $1,000. Thus, as a public policy issue, costs and access are important and interrelated.

The third related concept is quality of care. Again, quality is a question we would ask about any type of service or even a specific product to be purchased. Is it a quality product, or is the care I will receive of high quality? Is it at least of acceptable quality? For consumer products, we often trade off between quality and cost. People decide to accept a less well made product (one that may not last as long) if the price is lower. Once we begin to talk about a service such as healthcare, which involves the person's body and possible life or death consequences, the willingness of many people to accept tradeoffs between cost and quality is often low. Many people adopt the attitude that only the best quality is acceptable. In healthcare, experts discuss how everyone feels they deserve the best and most advanced care, even if they would not make the same choice about other goods and services. But what is the best quality? Are we always able to measure quality in healthcare? Consider an analogy to other service areas in American society. While even the wealthiest people often eat fast food sometimes and dine in elegant restaurants other times, most people want elegant, outstanding healthcare all the time, not "fast-food" healthcare. Issues of quality are very important and quickly become interwoven with policies about cost and access. That the government and individuals should not pay for healthcare of inferior quality is a statement that almost everyone agrees with. But must everyone have the most technologically sophisticated care for it to be of high quality? The phrases "two-tiered" and "two-class" system of care were often used in the past to describe aspects of U.S. healthcare, with one tier or class for individually (and insured) paying patients and another for charity (or more recently, government-funded) patients. Providing different levels of "quality" of care is generally no longer viewed as appropriate, unless all of it is at a minimum standard of quality. Clearly, quality becomes a third major consideration, along with cost and access.

Health Policy Formulation and the Role of Government in Healthcare Reform

Healthcare reform is one part of U.S. health policy that has occupied an important place in the country's domestic policy agenda, and its importance within that agenda has been growing over the past 35 years. A nation's health policy is part of its overall social policy. Given that, health policy formulation is influenced by the variety of social and economic factors that impact social policy development. Generally, policies are authoritative decisions made in the legislative, executive, or judicial branch of government that are intended to influence the actions, behaviors, or decisions of others. If a policy relates to improvement of health, having enough healthcare professionals, or issues such as cost, quality, and access of healthcare services, it is a part of healthcare policy. In the United States today, the government plays a major role in planning, directing, and financing healthcare services, although this was less true in earlier time periods (Kronenfeld 1997). Compared to some countries in the world, the United States has a complicated system of government that makes policy formulation and passage of subsequent enabling legislation difficult, not only in health but in other policy areas as well. The United States has a federal system of government that was created by the U.S. Constitution. At the time of the founding of the country in the 1790s, federalism was a legal concept that defined the constitutional division of authority between the federal government and the states. Federalism stressed the independence of each level of government from the other, while also incorporating certain functions (especially foreign policy) that were the exclusive area for the central (federal) government. Other policy areas, including healthcare, were initially conceived of as being left to the states.

While an expanded role for the federal government in many areas has become an accepted aspect of the way government works in the United States today, with much of the expansion of domestic programs beginning with the New Deal programs of the 1930s, the complexity of a federal system still creates some complications in how health programs operate. Certain health programs are joint federal-state efforts. One of the biggest and best known examples of this is the Medicaid program, which provides healthcare coverage for many lower-income Americans. Because this is a shared program in which both federal and state funds are used, but for which states must meet certain federal government requirements, differences can occur between the two units of government. A cutback or an increase in mandated eligibility at the federal level may cause a state to have to adjust its budget (Lee and Benjamin 1999). Meeting the state's share of the program can be difficult for states in times of declining state revenues, such as the recession in the United States that followed the 9/11 terrorist attacks. In fact, the continued economic recession in the first half of 2003 even led to some discussion in state legislatures about whether certain states would be able to provide the needed funds to continue to participate in Medicaid. Over the past few decades, as eligibility for Medicaid has been expanded at certain points, states have had to find the dollars in their budgets to match federal expenditures. These Medicaid match dollars have become one of the more rapidly rising portions of expenditures for states. These complexities can become one part of a push from states for the federal government to become a major player in and leader of healthcare reform efforts.

In addition to the complexity the federal system creates across levels of government, government in the United States has other limitations as well. The U.S. Constitution contains notions of limited government because of fears of a strong central government when the document was written and the importance placed on protecting rights of individuals. Two important aspects that relate to these fears are the reserve clause and the creation of three branches of government. The reserve clause states that any powers not explicitly given to the federal government are reserved for the states, and this clause is the basis of the important role of states within the United States.

There are three branches of government in the United States: executive, legislative, and judicial. At least in theory, these are separate and equal in power. Although popular culture in the United States now exalts the executive branch, in the person of the president, to be more powerful than the other branches, in reality, the U.S. president is much less powerful than the heads of state under certain other political systems. As opposed to a parliamentary system of government such as in Great Britain where the head of the party in the parliament is the prime minister, the head of the executive branch in the United States (the president) is elected separately from the legislative branch (Congress), and different political parties can be represented in the different branches. Thus, at any point in time, it may be much more difficult for the president's suggested policies to be enacted into law because the president may represent a different political party from the party that controls Congress. This can be made even more difficult because Congress has two different legislative bodies: the House of Representatives and the Senate. At any given time, each congressional body can have a different majority party. In combination, this division of powers among units of government and among branches of government creates an institutional structure that makes reform policies and major policy changes more difficult. Under a parliamentary system, the prime minister can propose new polices and generally have those enacted into legislation because the prime minister's party also controls the legislative branch of government. Generally, this has been given as one (although not the only) explanation of why major reforms, including reforms in the healthcare delivery system, are so difficult to accomplish in the United States (Steinmo and Watts, 1995).

In addition, the presence of two different legislative bodies, the House of Representatives and the Senate, only compounds the difficulty of having health reform legislation enacted. This is not accidental. The creation of two legislative branches was part of a compromise between large and small states at the time of the writing of the Constitution. The House of Representatives was viewed as the branch that was closer to the people, and each representative is responsible to a small district. Districts in each state are created in proportion to the percentage of the population in the United States, so large states have many more representatives in the House than do small states. In contrast, each state has only two senators, and they represent the entire state. Until the twentieth century, Senators were not popularly elected; rather, they were appointed by the legislatures of the states. The two legislative bodies create a further opportunity for divided and weakened government; even if the party of the president wins a majority in one of the houses of the legislature, it still does not have a majority in both, thus making it more difficult for new legislation to be passed.

All of these structural factors in the basic operation of the government of the United States make it more difficult to have major policy changes enacted. Despite this, the role of the federal government in healthcare has expanded over the past several hundred years. There have been times change has occurred and other times change has appeared likely and then failed politically. These specifics are discussed in the rest of this chapter.

The Early Role of the Federal Government in Health and Healthcare and Early Healthcare Reform Efforts up to the End of World War II

In the 1700s through much of the 1800s, healthcare was more of a cottage industry than the major organized industry of major hospitals, medical settings, physicians, and the many other healthcare professionals that we see today. Before the American Revolution, there were almost no real hospitals, and training of physicians mostly occurred in England or elsewhere in Europe. Gradually, some major hospitals were founded that were generally run as charities for the poor and training locations for physicians. Some medical schools were created, and more came into existence in the second half of the nineteenth century, but quality of the training was often poor.

Early federal legislation focused on special groups for whom the federal government had special responsibilities. Most sources mark the beginning of federal involvement with healthcare with the Act for the Relief of Sick and Disabled Seamen in 1798, also referred to as the Merchant Marine Services Act of 1798. This act provided health services for men who served in the Merchant Marine services, and it served two purposes: to provide care for this important type of worker in the country and also to protect all other Americans from the dangers of diseases that these sailors might bring back into the country as they returned from foreign ports. Around the same time, some legislation was passed to impose quarantines on ships entering U.S. ports to prevent epidemics. In 1800, legislation was passed authorizing federal officials to cooperate with state and local authorities to enforce quarantine laws.

Because the role of the federal government in healthcare was very limited during this time period, what in general was happening with health needs of regular Americans? From 1800 to 1850, there was not a large industry related to the delivery of healthcare, and big hospitals were not found across the country. Even in the small number of major cities in the United States at that time, healthcare was very different from the twenty-first-century version of healthcare. Healthcare was much more of a small business at that time, with individual physicians setting up their own practices and negotiating fees with patients. Some experts have said medicine was first a domestic enterprise and then became a commercial enterprise. During this period, government had little to do with the private transactions between medical practitioners and their patients except for redressing negligence (malpractice) and guaranteeing the sanctity of contracts if a physician agreed to provide care for a group of patients (Starr 1982).

The Civil War was a major defining event in American history in many ways, including healthcare and the role of the federal government in healthcare. Changes in healthcare were slow and incremental in the period from 1865 to 1900. The federal government gradually became more active in many ways. Some of the initial activity and growth of the government was essential to the conduct of the war, such as raising an army.

The Morrill Act in 1862 initiated federal aid to the states. This act granted federal lands to each state and allowed the profits of those lands to be used for support of public institutions of higher education; these institutions hosted many programs in nursing, nutrition, and later, medicine. Just as important to healthcare policy was the beginning of the use of the general welfare clause of the U.S. Constitution to justify some federal actions. Today, that clause is the major justification for most federal involvement in healthcare, including most medical research, Medicare, Medicaid, and health training programs (Kronenfeld 1997).

In the Civil War and post–Civil War eras, events that brought greater government involvement in health included immigration growth. Due to the very large numbers of immigrants that started to come to the United States, public attitudes about immigration were changing. Earlier waves of immigrants came from England, Scotland, Germany, and Ireland; newer waves consisted of new groups from southern and eastern Europe, such as Italy, Poland, and Russia, Many Americans feared these people as dangerous strangers who spoke other languages and therefore might bring strange customs and strange conditions into the United States. A general fear of the spread of disease in the population developed, and health legislation was passed giving the surgeon general of the Marine Services Hospitals the authority to impose quarantines to prevent the spread of diseases. The first general immigration law, passed in 1882, included provisions that allowed for the exclusion of immigrants for medical reasons. As part of this legislation, federal inspectors and physicians were allowed to go onto ships to check for diseases.

States and cities began to establish departments of public health, often to deal with the growth of cities due to both foreign immigration and internal mobility. By 1902, a health act was passed that clarified some federal health functions by renaming the Marine Hospital Services the Public Health and Marine Services and setting up a system of communication between state, territorial, and federal health officials. The surgeon general, the administrative head of the Public Health Service, was authorized to have an annual meeting of state and territorial health officers to discuss major health policies, issues, and concerns of the day. Early concerns were the control of trachoma (an eye disease) and typhoid fever (a highly infections disease transmitted by contaminated food and water), and nutritional deficiency diseases such as pellagra (caused by a lack of niacin in the diet).

By the early 1900s, some additional major health policy issues were being raised. Fueled by the investigative journalism that examined corruption in the production of drugs and foodstuffs, and by the success of novels that focused on this topic (such as *The Jungle* by Upton Sinclair) that focused on lack of sanitation in meat processing factories, reformers pushed for a greater role for the federal government in food and drug safety. These concerns resulted in the passage of the Federal Food and Drug Act of 1906. Initially, this legislation focused on regulations about adulteration and misbranding of food and drugs as well as control of substances within these products. This act has become the basis for most present-day regulation of testing, marketing, and promoting both prescription and over-the-counter medication. Issues related to this topic continue into the present, with some examples being whether tobacco can be considered a drug under this act and whether herbal food supplements need to be considered drugs under federal law to ensure their purity and content.

Within medicine itself, between 1900 and 1920 was a period of major intellectual ferment. Medicine was changing into a science-based field, but American medical education lagged behind the better renowned, scientifically based medical schools in Germany, Scotland, and England. Around 1900, the opening of a new medical school at John Hopkins University in Baltimore, Maryland, was a very conscious attempt to bring German-style medical education to the United States. That model of education was based on the application of some of the new scientific findings about germs as a cause of disease, about the role of vitamins in health and illness, and an understanding that physicians themselves could be the source of additional illnesses in patients if they did not pay attention to cleanliness and not spreading germs from one patient to another. Both a committee within the American Medical Association and Abraham Flexner, who conducted a study of medical education funded by the Carnegie Foundation for the Advancement of Teaching in 1910, ended up agreeing that medical education in the United States needed radical reform. The Flexner Report concluded that the training of physicians needed to become a university function, using a firm scientific foundation with full-time physicians as teachers, and that a bachelor's degree with an undergraduate science foundation needed to become the requirement to enter medical school. Over the next 30 years, the number of medical schools decreased substantially, and standards rose. Nursing education also began to focus on the provision of some scientific basis for its work, rather than just being an on-the-job training program. Hospitals, once seen as a place to send people to die who did not have the means to be able to die comfortably at home, also began to change in the early 1900s. As more technology was being developed, such as the use of x-ray machines, it became concentrated in hospitals. Gradually, people of all social classes became willing first to use hospitals and eventually to view the hospital as the preferred site for advanced care. These changes all led to a greater interest in the use of healthcare services, which then eventually raised more modern concerns about who is able to obtain those services and how the costs of those services can be paid.

These major reforms in medical education at the beginning of the twentieth century were centered in more urban areas. In frontier settings, most care was traditionally provided at home, by self-taught family members with the use of home remedy books. As immigration increased, the size of cities in the United States grew, and the frontier disappeared, the use of formal healthcare grew. Gradually, the issue of how to pay for this care arose. In some employment settings with high injury rates (such as mining), there was a push to create special healthcare insurance or access for workers, but up to (and in many cases, beyond) the beginning of the twentieth century, most Americans managed to pay for healthcare as part of usual life expenses.

The first major attempt to pass some type of health reform legislation and healthcare coverage was made during the presidency of Theodore Roosevelt. By the beginning of the twentieth century, concerns were beginning to be raised about access to healthcare services and coverage for workers who were too sick to go to work. Some countries in Europe were discussing making healthcare services available more widely to their populations. These discussions began to be picked up within the United States. While many groups in the United States were pushing for various types of reform, one of the most important was the American Association for Labor. This group tried to stimulate health insurance programs through state governments and labor unions, and it pushed for trying options such as sickness funds, as were being used in Germany in the early 1900s. Despite the early discussion of these topics, none of the proposed social changes led to any national legislation.

Conflict over World War I led to discrimination against German-based ideas, and sickness funds became viewed as "too German" a solution for America. Labor unions focused more on recruitment and their own growth, and less on broader social programs and goals, especially in the period after World War I when the United States entered a more conservative political era and labor unions felt threatened. In addition, pushing for a greater role for government in the provision of healthcare services became more difficult during the 1920s, as suspicions of "socialist" programs grew, and they increasingly viewed as "un-American."

Healthcare Reform and Federal Efforts during the Period between World War I and World War II, Including the Great Depression, and during World War II and the Immediate Postwar Era

Despite the increased conservatism mentioned earlier in this discussion in the period following World War I in the United States, there were a few notable pieces of legislation passed in this time frame. One of these was the Maternity and Infancy Act, also known as the Sheppard-Towner Act, which was passed in 1921. This legislation provided grants to states to help them develop health services for mothers and their children. While the goal of this program may seem simple and straightforward today, at the time, the program was very controversial. It generated criticism from the American Medical Association (AMA), which described it as "an imported socialistic scheme." The act also specified that the services had to be available to *all* residents of a state, regardless of race. This provision was very controversial in the 1920s, given the reality of race-based discrimination in programs in many states.

The essential design of the program became a very important predecessor to later federal efforts in health. The idea of providing grants to states for health programs has served as a prototype for federal grants-in-aid programs. This early and successful effort expanded the role of the federal government in the area of health. However, both the goals and the approach of this program became controversial in the 1920s. Critics were opposed to government involvement in the provision of healthcare services to people, arguing that it was a move toward socialism. In addition to that concern, some in the AMA had more pragmatic concerns about limitations on the pay of physicians and the continuation of physicians as "independent businessmen." The criticism was so significant and the commitment to the program by the political powers of the time so limited that the act was not renewed in 1929, and the program ceased to exist, although some of the functions of this legislation were later restored as part of the Social Security Act of 1935 (Skocpol 1992; Wallace Gold 1982).

In addition to this type of program for a specialized population group, the need for better access to healthcare services for the working population was a continued topic of discussion. Concern about economic insecurity grew in the 1930s as the Great Depression began and the economic situation of many average Americans worsened. President Franklin Roosevelt created the advisory Committee on Economic Security, which broached the idea of a government health insurance program. There were initial discussions of passing a Medicare-type program as part of New Deal reforms, but these early efforts never resulted in any provisions for health insurance being presented to Congress. Although the idea of provision of healthcare insurance for older adults was brought up, it was not included as part of Social Security legislation because of opposition from the American Medical Association. Roosevelt wanted to be sure that the essential Social Security legislation creating an old age pension system was enacted; when it became clear that the healthcare provision could potentially threaten passage of the overall Social Security legislation, he quickly backed off from it.

Although major health reform legislation was not passed during this era, the Great Depression did lead to major federal actions in a number of areas, including banking, employment patterns in the federal government, business regulation, and the creation of the Social Security system. The Social Security legislation created a social insurance program to provide economic security to older adults and marked the initiation of a means-tested social assistance program in the United States. Between 1935 and the 1970s, the welfare state expanded to include benefits for spouses and widows (1937), disability insurance for workers of all ages unable due to health concerns to work (1965), and Medicare and Medicaid (which will be discussed in more detail later in this chapter) (Quadagno 2004, 2005).

In addition to these individually based benefits, the Social Security Act of 1935 included a section (Title V) that authorized grants to the states for maternal and child health services, child welfare services, and services to "crippled" children. Another section (Title VI) authorized annual federal grants to states for investigating the problems of disease and sanitation, which led to the creation of new local health departments in many states and significantly increased overall federal assistance for state and local public health programs. By the end of fiscal year 1936, about 175 new local health departments had been created as part of this legislation (Kronenfeld 1997).

The program for crippled children represented a new thrust in federal legislation, as it included demonstration money that became the foundation of experience for amendments in later legislation that covered innovative program grants. The program included both comprehensive and preventive aspects, and covered all related medical care costs for children with physical disabilities or disabling conditions. While this was a small, specialized group in the population, the effort did represent the beginning of the federal government providing funds for direct care for a specialized group of the general population, not a group entitled to services due to occupation and service to the country (e.g., being on active duty in the military, being a wounded veteran of a war, or being in the merchant marine service).

Although some limited efforts to provide services to seriously disabled veterans had begun at the end of World War I, the Veterans Act of 1924 codified and extended the role of the federal government in the provision of healthcare services to veterans. That act extended medical care to veterans not only for treatment of disabilities associated with military service but also for other conditions requiring hospitalization. Preference was given to veterans who could not afford private care. In 1930, the Veterans' Administration was created as an independent federal agency to handle disabled soldiers and other veteran-related matters such as pensions. The activities of this agency were expanded greatly by the end of World War II, as the agency had to meet the needs of a much larger population of returning soldiers at the end of that war.

The federal government led the way in other areas related to health and protection of the health of the public during this era. Consumer protection in the drug arena was expanded by the passage in 1938 of the Food, Drug, and Cosmetic Act, which required manufacturers to demonstrate the safety of drugs before marketing them. The role of the federal government in research was expanded through the Ransdell Act of 1930, which created the National Institute of Health from the U.S. Health Service Hygienic Laboratory that had been established in 1901. The act provided money for buildings to house research activities, created a system of health fellowships, and authorized the acceptance of public donations for research on the cause, prevention, and cure of disease (Strickland 1978).

This role expanded in 1937 with the creation of the National Cancer Institute, which was authorized to award grants to non-governmental scientists and institutions, to provide fellowships for the training of scientists, and to fund direct federal government cancer research. Given the importance of health research in today's healthcare system, and the important role of the National Institutes of Health as one of the leading funders of health-related research in the world today, it is hard to overemphasize the importance of these acts.

As part of an overall administrative reorganization of the federal bureaucracy, the Roosevelt administration was interested in consolidating federal health functions. In 1939, the Public Health Service became a component of the Federal Security Agency (FSA). The Public Health Service Act, passed in 1944, created the Office of the Surgeon General, the National Institutes of Health, and bureaus of medical services and state services. The new federal agencies' activities included research and investigation into selected diseases and health problems, working with state and local health agencies to collect vital statistics (records on births, deaths, and other life events), and special grants for the major diseases of the time, such as venereal disease and tuberculosis control.

The Hill-Burton legislation (also known as the Hospital Survey and Construction Act of 1946) was the first major amendment to the Public Health Service Act. In the post–World War II era, many European countries passed legislation to reform their healthcare systems as a reward to the general population for the toil of over five years of warfare on the European continent, as a way to address concerns about social equity, and as a way to deal with the lack of attention given to civilian needs during wartime. There were still many similar concerns in the United States, even though the war itself had not occurred on U.S. soil and U.S. cities were not destroyed. Very little hospital construction occurred during the Great Depression and World War II. In the Great Depression, the lack of funds and the overall bad economy meant private hospitals (generally owned by physicians) were not built, nor did municipalities and counties have funds available to build new city and county hospitals. Once World War II started, building materials were saved for the war effort, and little new civilian construction of any type occurred, including hospitals.

In addition to the pent-up demand for newer buildings and facilities, there was also a belief that more people would be interested in using hospital and physician services by the late 1940s. Medical technology was improving, and the place to access the new technology in the U.S. healthcare system at that time was hospitals. During World War II, many soldiers received health services through the federal government. Also, many laborers had received health insurance benefits in lieu of raises during the war, as providing health insurance was one way to reward workers during a period when salary increases were controlled by the federal government. The negative image of hospitals as a place for people to die and for people with no other options for care continued to decline.

Within the United States, then, as in many European countries after the end of World War II, debate began about a more comprehensive national health insurance system. President Truman revived this discussion in 1945, and he, along with the more liberal wing of the Democratic Party, promoted national health insurance legislation. Organized labor, a major supporter of the Democratic Party at that time, was also in favor of more comprehensive healthcare reform. Some of the major support groups assumed significant reform was likely; however, the AMA and several important business interests became vocal opponents of major reform. The AMA launched a major national education campaign to try to prevent the passage of national health insurance legislation and instead to promote private health insurance. At that time, the basic structure of the AMA was the county medical society. If a physician was not a member of the county medical society, he could not be a member of the state organization or obtain staff privileges at most hospitals. The AMA national headquarters charged a

$25 fee to all members and used those funds for the fight against the Truman–liberal Democratic plan. Speeches, pamphlets, cartoons, and other kinds of publicity materials were sent to county and state groups, all with the goal of making the public hostile to national health insurance. The message included the idea that national health insurance was socialized medicine and part of a communist plot to destroy freedom in the United States (Quadagno 2004).

The AMA joined forces with some important and powerful employer and insurer groups such as the Blue Cross Association, the American Hospital Association, pharmaceutical and drug manufacturers, and the Chamber of Commerce. These groups took a public position of opposition to national health insurance and endorsed private health insurance. These campaigns affected public opinion, and although 1945 polls showed 75 percent of Americans supported national health insurance, by 1949, support had declined to only 21 percent (Quadagno 2004).

Although everyone recognized the need to increase the involvement of the federal government in healthcare and in meeting unmet healthcare needs, neither the Republicans nor the moderate wing of the Democratic Party were in favor of national health insurance. As a compromise once more comprehensive legislation was not passed, Senator Lister Hill of Alabama devised the strategy of having the government provide funds for hospital construction, with the assumption that the private marketplace would be able to meet the less expensive needs of provision of health insurance. The Hill-Burton Act became the major postwar initiative of the federal government.

The act provided grants to allow states to inventory their existing hospitals and health centers, and to survey the need for the construction of additional health facilities. After state surveys were completed, grants for hospital construction were made available. Funds for surveys and planning were allocated to the states based on total state population; federal funding covered up to a third of the total costs. Funds for construction were allocated through a formula based on population and per capita income, and again covered up to a third of the costs.

Among strategists for health insurance, the level of controversy over compulsory health insurance became a problem. People such as Wilbur J. Cohen and Isadore S. Falk, who were very involved in the early drafting of both the Social Security health insurance proposals and Truman's health insurance proposals, started to think of other strategies. Cohen and Falk served as advisers to Federal Security Agency administrator Oscar Ewing. Together, they came up with the idea of supporting more modest, narrower proposals. They decided that a plan more likely to pass Congress was one that would provide federal health insurance to beneficiaries of Social Security payments as part of the Old Age and Survivors Insurance. In June 1951, Ewing announced a limited proposal to provide 60 days of health insurance each year to the then 7 million retirees receiving Social Security benefits, but this did not pass.

The decision to shift to a plan focused on older adults (Medicare) was a political, pragmatic one. In a comparative context, it was unusual because most other industrial nations had not begun their programs with older adults. More typical was the coverage of low-income workers, but this involved means tests, which was a strategy avoided in the United States due to stigma. Many policy analysts and political scientists have pointed out that in the United States, rather than having very large major public policy shifts, changes in public policy often come in small increments. The shift to a focus on older adults reflects the success of this incremental approach in the United States.

According to two researchers who have studied the debates around the creation of Medicare, Marmor (2000) and Oberlander (2003), there were four major objections to Truman's health plan. First, general medical insurance would be a "giveaway" program and would not distinguish between the deserving and undeserving poor. Second, it would aid too many wealthy or well-off Americans who did not need help.

Third, utilization of existing medical services would grow too rapidly and exceed the capacity of the system. Finally, there would be excessive federal control of physicians, which could provide a precedent for socialism in the United States. To get around these objections, the idea of a program limited to older adults was attractive. The concern about a giveaway program was diminished because older adults were seen as a group that was, on average, poorer, sicker, and less likely to be insured than other Americans. In addition, older adults garnered public sympathy as a group, and the issue that a person should simply earn more money to pay for services was not a relevant consideration. By this time in the United States, many people were receiving health insurance through the workplace, but as people grew older and retired, they lost this insurance, making the restriction to older adults a logical one based on the way health insurance was growing in the United States.

The decision to tie a program to the existing Social Security system made sense based on the widespread support that Social Security had gained among the public. The system was seen not as a welfare benefit but as an earned benefit of retired workers, as it was provided to people who had paid into the system through payroll taxes in their working years. This idea that the benefits had been earned was very important in gaining the support of the public for the program as not being a welfare program. Because it benefitted the majority of older adults, support could be gathered among a wide range of current workers, both as a benefit they would receive in the future and one that would benefit their parents more quickly. Thus, it was hoped, a shift to a program for older adults would gain broad political support.

In 1952, Eisenhower campaigned against socialized medicine, which for him included both the earlier Truman proposals and more modest proposals for health insurance for older adults. In addition, in 1952, the Republicans gained majorities in both the House of Representatives and the Senate, and there was a general conservative shift in the national political mood. Thus, during the Eisenhower administration (1952–1960), most Medicare bills, whatever the type, really had no chance of being enacted.

Eisenhower, Kennedy, and Johnson: Years of Expansion and Growing Federal Involvement in Health

While advocates of a government health insurance program realized that no major social legislation would pass during World War II due to large government expenses as part of the war effort, there was consensus within the more liberal elements of the Democratic Party that there should be a major push again for such a program after the war was over. Although national health insurance was the topic under discussion, many of proposed versions focused more on incremental Medicare-type legislation. This legislation did continue to be introduced into most sessions of Congress once World War II ended, but they had little chance of success in the late 1940s and 1950s. Even when the Democrats controlled the White House with Truman as president in 1948, the congressional majorities were not in place to support it. Most Republicans opposed it, as did more conservative Democrats. Even the Democratic majorities included segments of the party that were opposed to a government-funded healthcare program for older adults.

Although the 1950s were generally a more conservative era, they were not static. In 1954, the Democrats regained control of both houses of Congress, raising the chances of discussion of various social policy issues. However, the prospects for a Medicare-type proposal were not good, as the Democrats still did not have a programmatic majority capable of enacting federal health insurance for older adults. The leadership of both the House Ways and Means Committee and the Senate Finance Committee were resistant to a Medicare proposal, which, along with the absence of a president supportive of the legislation, made major political change unlikely.

Slowly, some change began to occur. In 1956, disability insurance for workers over the age of 50 was passed, an approach that was pushed by people such as Wilbur Cohen, director of research for the Social Security Administration, along with people who had been important in the Truman years in developing plans for national health insurance. They saw disability legislation as another incremental achievement that helped provide some greater security for older workers in the absence of national health insurance. In 1957, Representative Aime Forand, a Democrat from Rhode Island, proposed a bill on Medicare. Beginning in 1958, serious congressional interest in special health insurance programs for older adults began to grow. From 1958 to 1965, the congressional finance committees held annual hearings on the topic. In 1958, the Ways and Means Committee in the House held a hearing on the bill, but the new Democratic chair of the committee, Wilbur Mills from Arkansas, opposed the Forand bill, and it did not make it out of committee.

These hearings revitalized Medicare as a political issue and brought back the attention of the AMA, which believed it had defeated these ideas for good during the Truman administration. In response, the AMA raised its lobbying budget fivefold to increase its ability to criticize and raise opposition against the Forand bill. Bringing back arguments from the late 1940s, the AMA argued that the Forand bill would bring an unwelcome intrusion of the government into private medical practice. It also argued that older adults were better off than some other age groups, but the main thrust of the opposition was ideological. The AMA wanted to convince the public that health insurance for older adults would be the first step toward national socialism, and the group used code words of the time that were designed to raise political concerns and make many politicians reluctant to support the idea. The AMA also helped line up other opponents that had some focus on healthcare or insurance concerns (e.g., the American Hospital Association, the National Association of Blue Shield Plans, and the Life Insurance Association of America) as well as various business organizations (e.g., the National Association of

Manufacturers, the Chamber of Commerce, and the American Farm Bureau Federation). Given the ideological orientation of the opposition, groups such as the American Legion also opposed the legislation. Despite the hope among advocates of health insurance for older adults that a move to enact government health insurance only among older adults and tie it to the existing, and popular, Social Security program would dampen political opposition, this did not happen initially. The acrimonious debate that had occurred at the time of the Truman proposal reappeared, with similar proponents and opponents, and public attention was refocused on the issue as political commentators and the press began to follow parts of the debate. Among the proponents of the legislation were major labor groups (e.g., the AFL-CIO), health-related groups (e.g., the American Nurses Association, the National Association of Social Workers, and the American Geriatrics Society), and more liberal social action–oriented groups (e.g., the Council of Jewish Federations and Welfare Funds, the American Association of Retired Workers, and the National Farmers Union). Differences between the groups opposing and in favor of Medicare were often along the lines of their differences on other important political issues of the day, such as disability insurance and federal aid for education. Gradually, however, the shift to a focus on older adults and the creation of some lobby groups focused on older adults did begin to shift some of the terms of the debate.

A special Senate subcommittee on aging was created, under Democratic senator Pat McNamara from Michigan, and the group held a series of public meetings on the topic in 38 different cities between 1959 and 1961. This raised public awareness of issues of older adults generally, and especially the issue of health insurance for older adults. An interesting split occurred between the Forand Social Security approach and a welfare-oriented approach. The Social Security approach pushed to cover all older adults who were covered under Social Security, while a welfare approach advocated a focus on people over 65 whose own resources were inadequate to meet medical expenses. In terms of benefits, the Social Security approach covered hospitalization, nursing homes, and surgical coverage, while the welfare approach was broader and covered physicians' services, dental care, drugs, and hospital expenses. The Social Security approach proposed funding through additional Social Security taxes, a regressive approach that would take a greater percentage of money from workers who were paid less because at that time, there was a fairly low cap on the amount of wages taxed for Social Security (there is still a cap today on wages taxed for Social Security, but it is at a much higher level, and there is no longer a cap for Medicare, although there was such a cap initially). An advantage of this approach was the absence of any means test, which critics felt would be insulting to older adults. There was also an argument that the absence of a means test would broaden the political appeal of the program, as it would benefit all older adults. A welfare approach would use state matching funds along with federal income tax revenues, which is generally a more progressive source of taxation. The Social Security approach would lead to uniform national standards administered by the Social Security Administration, whereas a welfare approach would lead to varying standards administered by state and local officials.

Although the Eisenhower administration remained opposed to any legislation similar to the Forand bill, some Republicans, including the likely presidential candidate Richard Nixon, became worried that this opposition could be a detriment to a Republican presidential candidate. Some congressional conservatives, especially on the Democratic side, came up with a counterproposal, a bill sponsored by Senators Robert Kerr of Oklahoma and Wilbur Mills of Arkansas. This bill proposed expanding federal aid to states that were providing medical care assistance to poor older adults. The Kerr-Mills bill proposed federal matching grants of 50 to 80 percent of the costs to participating states. This was the welfare-oriented approach. By the time the bill was up for a vote in Congress, Democratic presidential candidate John F. Kennedy had decided to use medical care for older adults as one policy issue on which he could distinguish himself from Nixon, and this became a Democratic Party plank at the nominating convention. This raised the attention being paid to the Kerr-Mills bill, and the AMA decided to endorse the bill as a preferable alternative to Medicare itself. The legislation was passed by Congress and signed by President Eisenhower.

The victory was viewed differently by different groups. While conservatives viewed this as legislation passed as an alternative to Medicare, liberals viewed it as a first step toward a broader Medicare proposal. Despite some enthusiasm for the program when the legislation was passed, it was not very successful in practice. Although some experts had estimated that there were 2.4 million people on old-age assistance and 10 million medically indigent that could benefit from the program, some critics such as McNamara felt many of the states would never provide the matching funds needed to participate in the program. McNamara's predictions proved more accurate over time. Many states never participated in the program (32 of 50 by 1963), and by 1965, five large industrial states (California, New York, Massachusetts, Michigan, and Pennsylvania) were using almost 90 percent of the Kerr-Mill funds, even though those states had only a third of the older adult population in the United States. Not only was the geographic distribution of the recipients limited, but the range of benefits provided was also less than allowed by the program. In 1963, only four states provided the full range of care allowed for in the bill.

A Push for Medicare Legislation in the Kennedy Administration

As Senator John Kennedy decided to run in the 1960 presidential campaign, he made the passage of Medicare legislation an important part of his campaign. Kennedy's victory in that election meant that now there was presidential sponsorship for the Medicare legislation. In his first State of the Union address,

President Kennedy called for the enactment of healthcare provisions for older adults by the end of the year. He labeled his proposed new programs the New Frontier and included a variety of domestic proposals within it, one of which was health insurance for older adults. A new Medicare bill was introduced by Senator Clinton Anderson of New Mexico and Representative Cecil King of California. This bill provided 90 days of hospitalization coverage, 240 days of home health services, 180 days of nursing home care, and outpatient diagnostic services. It would extend these benefits to 14 million Americans over the age of 65 and would be financed by a 0.25 percent increase in Social Security taxes. The Kennedy administration pushed for this legislation with a public campaign that included a series of rallies and a nationally televised appeal in 1962. Fearful of the kind of opposition that had derailed a similar proposal in the Truman years, Kennedy stressed that this was not socialized medicine but rather prepayment for healthcare costs with freedom of choice of providers assured.

Despite the attempt to distance this new effort from the fears about the earlier Truman proposals, some of the same political issues that hindered Truman's push for national health insurance were problems for Kennedy. He lacked a firm programmatic majority in Congress and, as with Truman, was often frustrated by the conservative coalition of southern Democrats and Republicans in Congress. Among his own party's leadership, Ways and Means chair Wilbur Mills was concerned about the program and feared that the fiscal consequences would be bad for Social Security overall.

Moreover, the process for the selection of the Ways and Means Committee in the House worked against expansion of social welfare issues, including Medicare for older adults. Democrats on the Ways and Means Committee in that era also made up the Committee on Committees that made Democratic committee assignments. This ended up freezing the geographical distribution in the Ways and Means Committee with nine Democratic liberal members in a minority in terms of social policy expansions and with southern Democrats and some Republicans representing the opposition. If it was clear that the House would favor legislation, such legislation was reported out of committee and voted on by all members. However, if the senior members of this committee (especially the more conservative southern Democrats) felt that a bill would face a bitter, close floor fight, often the committee either did not report the bill out or wrote compromises into the legislation before it hit the floor of the House. Mills, whose own Kerr-Mills bill had just become law in the Eisenhower administration, was not initially inclined to be supportive. Moreover, it appeared that redistricting based on the 1960 census might cause Arkansas to lose two House seats and might result in a contested election in Mills's own district, reinforcing his more conservative tendencies because he was concerned about pressure in his home state in addition to broader national concerns. Because of these pressures and the pressure for Kennedy to achieve legislative success in other areas, such as his trade and tax legislation, the Medicare bill did not surface in 1961. No vote was even taken.

Some of the same opposing groups that had been the backbone of opposition to the Truman proposals became active against a new Medicare bill. The AMA led the opposition again, especially in terms of public advertisements and public comment. The group funded newspaper, radio, and television ads that again brought charges of socialism, arguing that a task force would enter the privacy of the examination room and eliminate the freedom of Americans to choose their own physicians and the freedom of physicians to treat patients as they saw fit. Beyond this national advertising, the AMA actively opposed the bill in many other ways. It sponsored reproductions of congressional speeches against the bill and distributed them in many American communities. The organization also enlisted county medical societies to provide speakers against the legislation in a variety of public forums. In addition, at the level of the individual physician, the AMA provided material and urged physicians to place that material in their reading areas for patients and to let patients know that their own physician opposed these changes and thought it would be bad for the patient.

Even though Democrats retained control of Congress following the 1962 elections, not much changed in terms of the committees controlling the introduction of legislation and the likelihood of passing some type of Medicare legislation. While various efforts to have votes taken on the legislation did occur, nothing passed. The chances of passage in 1963 were lower as Congress began to think about the elections in 1964, including the presidential election. It appeared as though a further push for Medicare would have to wait for Kennedy's second term, assuming he was successful in the 1964 elections. All these assumptions changed quickly. In November 1963, Kennedy's assassination changed many aspects of "politics as usual." Lyndon Johnson, Kennedy's vice president, took over as president and began to prepare to run for election on his own in 1964. The outcome of that election would be critical in determining the chances of Medicare's passage in the future.

The 1964 Election of LBJ and the Passage of Medicare

The 1964 election, which pitted the then-incumbent Democratic president Lyndon Baines Johnson (often known as LBJ) against Republican nominee Senator Barry Goldwater from Arizona, resulted in a very one-sided election that resulted in a landslide victory for the Democratic Party. Part of this was a reaction to the assassination of President Kennedy, which increased the popularity of the Democratic Party. In addition, Johnson was a skillful politician with many years of experience, and the campaign that Goldwater ran never captured the support of the American electorate. Given the large majorities, not only was LBJ elected, but the Democratic Party gained 32 seats in the House of Representatives, providing the party with a 2 to 1 ratio (295 Democratic seats to 140 Republican seats), the largest lead since New Deal days under FDR in the 1930s.

Similarly, the Senate margin was a large one for the Democratic Party, with 68 Democratic senators and only 32 Republican senators. One reading of Johnson's victory over Goldwater was that it provided support for what Johnson called his Great Society programs that included Medicare as one of the pieces of social legislation. Johnson campaigned for a variety of social reforms, including Medicare, and emerged from the election with control over both houses of Congress and a popular mandate for social change. The debate over legislation created a very specific type of program, so understanding the debate helps explain issues in Medicare's early decades and some of the problems leading up to the healthcare reform debates of today.

Given their large majorities, House Democrats were able to prevent delaying tactics for a variety of social legislation through modifications of House rules. Most importantly, the "21-day rule" was put back into place, meaning that bills could be discharged from the House Rules Committee after a maximum delay of three weeks (21 days). In addition to this rule change, the composition of the Ways and Means Committee was modified to better reflect the strength of the parties in the House as a whole instead of three majority and two minority members as in the past. This changed the composition of the committee in 1965 from 15 Democrats and 10 Republicans to 17 Democrats and 8 Republicans. These changes helped ensure passage of Medicare, and the issues and debates quickly became over what the actual legislation would include. In some ways, as other scholars have also noted (Oberlander 2003; Marmor 2000), this quick shift to a guaranteed success for the legislation left proponents somewhat unprepared as to whether a more comprehensive program might be the best approach. Instead, advocates continued to press for a more incremental program that emphasized maximizing consensus on a clearly defined, but somewhat minimal, set of benefits, leaving the issues of more comprehensive benefits as an area for future expansion. Medicare coverage as a basic aspect remained focused on 60 days of hospitalization and 60 days of nursing home care, with coverage for physician's bills an elective part of the program. Coverage was focused on older adults, and financing was to occur through a Social Security approach.

While Democrats quickly recognized how much the political circumstance had changed and what that meant, Republicans and other opponents of Medicare legislation (such as the AMA) only partially recognized just how much the political circumstances had changed. Republicans understood that passage of some type of Medicare legislation was now virtually inevitable and wanted to avoid being labeled as obstructionists. However, Republicans felt there was not much agreement on what a program should actually be and that this gave room for Republican criticism and opposition efforts. They focused on inadequate benefits, and some, such as Byrnes (the ranking Republican on the House Ways and Means Committee), proposed his own bill that would provide a voluntary program of federal payments to subsidize private health insurance for older adults. This would be a broader program, including physician bills and drug coverage, and general revenues would finance the program. As a group with grave concerns about what would actually be in the legislation, the AMA came up with a separate proposal of its own, called Eldercare. This program was to be implemented by states but would include hospital and physician coverage, as well as coverage of surgical fees, drug costs, nursing home costs, and services such as x-rays and laboratory charges. By February 1965, three different proposals were before the Congress: the King-Anderson bill, the Byrnes Republican proposal, and the AMA Eldercare proposal.

The most likely outcome, given the strength of the Democratic party majorities, was that Congress would move forward toward passage of the administration's bill (HR and S 1, the King-Anderson bill). As early as January, hearings were being held, as were executive sessions in private, which often indicate serious movement toward passage of legislation in Congress. The AMA, given its major concerns, testified at

the hearings. As when this type of legislation had been proposed in the past, the organization again raised concerns about
socialized medicine. This was irritating to the committee members, and Chairman Mills ended up refusing to consult AMA
representatives as the hearings and deliberations continued.

By March, hearings were also planned on the Byrnes
Republican bill. By this time, almost everyone agreed that
something was likely to pass, and Republicans wanted to prevent the Democrats from taking all the credit for passage of
Medicare legislation. They also began to publicize the inad-
equacies of the Democratic bill. Byrnes emphasized the major
areas of health costs not covered by the Democratic proposal,
such as physicians' bills and drug costs. Byrnes argued that one
major advantage of his bill was that it was voluntary, with older
adults free to decide whether to join. Even though the AMA
was publicizing and pushing its own Eldercare plan and discussing and publicizing the problems with the Democratic bill, most
of the discussion in the House was about the Byrnes proposal, not
Eldercare. The Byrnes and Democratic proposals were being
presented as mutually exclusive alternatives.

In early March, Mills started discussing some ways to com-
bine aspects of each proposal, which was somewhat of a surprise
move. Up to that point in time, the head of the Department of
Health, Education, and Welfare (DHEW), Wilbur Cohen, had
mentioned a three-pronged approach: the hospital program of
HR 1 first, then private health insurance for physician's coverage, and an expanded Kerr-Mills program as a safety-net type
of program for the indigent among older adults. Although there
had initially been some hesitancy on the Democratic side that
Mills was trying to scuttle the entire effort, Cohen became convinced this was not true. Cohen convinced the Democrats that
Mills's strategy was really a way to expand HR 1, based on
some of the criticisms of the Republicans. Byrnes initially was
not enthusiastic about this approach and wanted to see his
own approach seriously considered, but the House Ways and
Means Committee in March concentrated on working out

some of the combinations that might be possible. Payments for drugs outside of hospitals and nursing homes ended up being rejected for fear of costs being too high, for example, and such coverage was not part of most work-based healthcare policies at the time. Some aspects of Byrnes's financing approach received positive comments, and individual premium payments by current Social Security recipients for physician services were adopted. Many, many technical issues arose that later became important in Medicare, such as how to pay hospital-based specialists such as anesthesiologists, pathologists, and radiologists. Groups such as Blue Cross and the American Hospital Association became more actively involved in helping to draft parts of the legislation and in answering technical questions about hospital benefits. The Medicare Bill reported to the House on March 29, 1965, included parts of the original administration bill, parts of the Byrnes benefit package, and AMA's suggestion of an expanded Kerr-Mills program. As the legislation developed, these features became part of two different amendments to the existing Social Security legislation: Title 18, which included the hospital insurance program and some of the Byrnes extensions to cover voluntary physician's insurance, and Title 19, an expanded Kerr-Mills program that became known as Medicaid and became an addition to the initial Medicare proposal, rather than a substitute as the AMA had originally suggested. Despite including some Republican suggestions, in the final vote of the committee, there was a straight party vote of 17 in favor and 8 opposed.

The House met to vote on the legislation, now quite long (296 pages), and members gave Mills a standing ovation for his work on drafting this legislation through the committee. Byrnes was provided with a chance to present his alternative bill, and some Democrats actually favored that option, but the idea of sending that version forward was defeated. Instead, the committee bill (now HR 6675) was passed, largely on party lines. Because at the time the Senate was viewed as the more liberal of the legislative bodies, there was little concern that something would pass there, although, as is usual during the legislative process, there were questions about specific details. Two questions that became important were whether the method of paying inhospital specialists would remain, and whether there might be a move to make the program more generous, perhaps by varying the hospital deductible according to beneficiaries' income. The Senate version did contain a different payment plan for the inhospital specialists, one the AMA vehemently opposed and felt was much worse than the version in the House legislation. The Senate version also included unlimited hospital care with a coinsurance provision.

After each house of Congress had passed its own version, as is typically the case, the legislation had to go to a conference committee (a standard practice to resolve differences between the details of a bill passed in the House of Representatives and the version passed in the Senate). The House version of paying inhospital specialists became final in the bill. Most final points were compromises between the House and the Senate. On benefit duration, the more generous Senate version had allowed unlimited days and the House version 60 days, while the final version allowed 60 days with the $40 House deductible and an additional 30 days with the Senate $10 coinsurance provision. On skilled nursing home coverage, the House had provided 20 days and 2 more days for each unused hospital day up to a maximum of 100. The Senate had allowed 100 days with a copay of $5 a day for each day over 20, which became the conference version. The less generous House allowance of 100 posthospital home health days became the final version. Senate versions of details on outpatient diagnostic services and psychiatric coverage became the conference report version. This revised conference version was passed by the House on July 27 and by the Senate two days later, leading to the triumphant signing ceremony in Independence, Missouri (to honor former president Truman and his initial push for this type of legislation), on July 30, 1965.

Issues in the U.S. Healthcare System after Passage of Medicare and Medicaid

Once Medicare and Medicaid had passed, issues began to emerge. First, Medicare and Medicaid provided care for only some portions of the U.S. population—older adults and poor people. Even within that focus, issues quickly arose about implementation and costs. Many of these issues and concerns set the stage for today's issues. To bring older adults into the mainstream of American medicine, the program ended up looking very similar to decent health insurance coverage for typical Americans in regards to benefits, reimbursement structures, and administrative aspects. Medicare resembled typical Blue Cross–Blue Shield coverage at that time, with an emphasis on coverage for acute illness, generous payments to physicians and hospitals, and little oversight. Thus, older adults received much greater access to healthcare services, and the medical profession was reassured that the federal government would not disrupt the ways in which the healthcare system operated.

Over time, many aspects of the program changed. The good coverage of the 1960s became problematic coverage as private health insurance changed more easily and rapidly than did Medicare. The expectation that Medicare would take care of most of the healthcare needs of older adults with little out of pocket expenses was not really met (nor, in some ways, were those expectations realistic even at the very beginning of the program). The lack of oversight led to high costs, which eventually led to reorganization of reimbursement approaches for both hospitals and physicians, which led to the federal government changing the ways in which the healthcare system operated. Over time, the attempt to find ways to hold down costs became very important.

Another basic assumption was that Medicare would provide all people age 65 and older with the same health insurance coverage. Whatever a person's income level before retirement, or after retirement, everyone would participate in the same program and would have the same benefits, premiums, and cost-sharing requirements. A high-income person with a large pension in addition to Social Security and income from investments would not pay more for Medicare than a person whose only source of income was Social Security. One positive aspect of this situation in the early years of Medicare was strong support for Medicare across all older adults because everyone received similar benefits. In 1965, one reason for treating all people the same was the principle of universalism, which led to the assumption that all citizens should receive certain basic benefits. There was also the public image that older adults were a poorer and more dependent segment of the population and therefore deserved government assistance. While this assumption was largely accurate in 1965, it has become less so over time. Since then, changes have occurred not so much in benefits, but in the basic payments that are charged for people to participate in some aspects of Medicare.

Another expectation was that Medicare signaled the government's assumption of a role in health insurance, perhaps even a first step toward a more universal health insurance system. The architects of the initial legislation and early administrators, such as Robert Ball, a commissioner of the Social Security Administration, stated that insurance for older adults was a fallback position from more comprehensive reform. Expansions were expected, perhaps by age group to cover all children or to cover broader population groups. Many at the time expected a push for more changes and expansions in the system fairly quickly, but this did not occur. Parts of Medicare and Medicaid have been expanded, and SCHIP (the state child health insurance program) was created, but Medicare has remained the major federally administered health insurance program, with benefits restricted to older adults and people with disabilities. Debates continue over major changes in health insurance coverage in the United States.

One final expectation related to the 1965 program was that Medicare would be a system of public health insurance, guided by the federal government. Using some of today's language in healthcare debates, Medicare was a single-payer program, not a subsidized private health insurance program. This became the basic structure of the program despite the desires of the health insurance companies and many physicians to have a subsidized health insurance program. Many believe this occurred because private health insurance and the marketplace were already viewed as having failed in the provision of health insurance coverage to older adults; thus, government action was required. Over time, the basic aspects of Medicare changed in many ways, and some of these changes will be covered later in this chapter.

The First Five Years of Medicare and Medicaid

While the joy over passage of Medicare was intense in July 1965, the complex realities of putting into place and managing such a large program began to emerge as implementation began. The year between passage and implementation of the program (on July 1, 1966) was very busy, both in public and behind the scenes. Publicly, there were major tasks of informing the public and making sure that people 65 of age and older understood some things about the new program and their rights related to coverage and benefits under the program.

The initial creation of Medicare was complex partially because of the two different initial aspects of the program: Part A, the hospital insurance component (or HI), covers certain amounts of inpatient hospital care, home care, hospice care, and care in a skilled nursing facility; and Part B covers physician services. Part A is financed by a compulsory matching payroll tax; Part B is the supplementary health insurance portion, sometimes known as SMI or supplementary medical insurance. Beneficiaries pay a premium for Part B each month, which is generally deducted from their Social Security payments.

One of the more challenging aspects of implementation was ensuring people understood the need to actually enroll in the

Part B portion of Medicare. People had to sign up and agree to have a $3 monthly payment withheld from their Social Security check. The Social Security Administration began a large public service campaign, using both national and local media sources, to inform the public, especially older adults, about the new program. In addition, older adults on public assistance needed to be informed of the slightly different ways in which they would participate in the program. Over half of the states took responsibility for informing this group of citizens of the details of the new program as it would apply to them.

While these were massive tasks, they were generally completed successfully. By the end of the first year of Medicare implementation, 93 percent of older adults (about 19 million people) had enrolled in Part B. Usage of the program rapidly grew. By the end of the first year of operation, one in five older adults had used their Medicare benefits for hospital care, and 12 million had used their Part B services. On average that first year, Medicare paid about 80 percent of hospital expenses for this group.

Less visible to the public, but just as important as letting people know about the new program, was the task of evaluating healthcare facilities whose bills could be paid by the new program (hospitals, nursing homes, and home health agencies). The new law required that facilities had to agree to participate in the new program and that they had to meet a variety of specified conditions, including meeting standards of care and providing services on a nondiscriminatory basis in compliance with the Civil Rights Act of 1964. This latter requirement was especially difficult in some portions of the South, and, in reality, there were hospitals in the South that received program payments during the first year of operation but did not completely meet this requirement. Operationally, however, one of the early concerns was to ensure Medicare benefits were not denied to older adults who happened to live in formerly segregated areas of the southern United States.

There were some early implementation problems, perhaps not unexpected in the beginning of a massive new government program. Payments to providers were sometimes delayed, especially during the first summer of operation. Fears about hospital overcrowding were not realized. While not all physicians complied, overall, the physician participation rate was good, and the president of the American Medical Association at the time, James Appel, was helpful in urging physicians to cooperate (at one time, there had been talk of a physician boycott). The organization provided consultations about how to participate, leading to high physician utilization rates.

There is a certain irony about the ways that Medicare benefitted physicians. Physicians, through the American Medical Association, were among the most hostile critics of Medicare prior to its passage, arguing that it would destroy the strength and operation of physician services in the United States. Actually, physicians initially received substantial income supplements from Medicare, and most physicians ended up being reimbursed for services they often provided for free or at a reduced cost to older adults prior to the creation of Medicare.

At the time of passage, most experts agreed that the new program would help fund hospitals because older adults would be better able to pay their hospital bills, and it would also help insurance companies, who no longer would be pressured to provide affordable health insurance to older adults, a group whose costs insurers argued was too difficult to predict. Physicians' improved abilities to collect fees did not receive much discussion or attention prior to passage of the legislation; nevertheless, this was a benefit in the early years of implementation.

Much of what happened in the first years of the operation of Medicare was partially expected, but both the total amount of utilization and the costs became an issue. For a variety of reasons, costs ended up being higher than expected. One explanation is that both hospital and physician fees rose, partially because the arrangements for paying physicians were quite generous. There are estimates that physician fees initially rose 5 to 8 percent, and physician incomes went up 11 percent (Marmor 2000). Partially, the method by which both physicians and hospitals were paid became an issue for Medicare. There was no specific limit set on what a physician could charge. Instead, physicians were allowed to be paid reasonable charges—defined as customary for the individual physician and no higher than charges generally prevailing locally or regularly paid by Medicare's program administrators (generally, Blue Cross for hospital expenses and Blue Shield for Part B physician expenses). There was an expectation that physicians would charge more than they had collected from some poor, older adult patients, as this was not viewed as a charity program, and there was a concern that patients with Medicare benefits should not be treated as charity cases. As the first year began, however, it became clear that there was really no agreement either among physicians or the government about what the upper limit should be for "prevailing charges," nor was there much preexisting knowledge about what physicians were actually charging. Medicare began with an open-ended method of paying physicians, and concerns grew among physicians that there would be codification and freezing of physician fees by the fiscal intermediaries. Similarly, concerns grew among government officials that costs would be much higher than initial estimates.

Similar problems, perhaps even more serious, existed in the area of hospital prices. The Labor Department's consumer price survey showed that the average daily service charge in American hospitals increased 21.9 percent in the first year of Medicare's operation. By the summer of 1967, it was clear to the Johnson administration that this could be a very big problem, and the secretary of the Department of Health, Education and Welfare, John Gardner, was given the task of studying the reasons behind the large increase. The report pointed out that in requiring hospitals to reexamine their costs and charges initially, many hospitals increased their charges. Although hospital costs continued to increase in the second year of the program, the rate of increase was not as large in the second year. Other factors continued to push increases in costs. Allowances for depreciation and capital costs were taken into account in the determination of hospital reimbursement rates, and this created a built-in inflation push. In 1968 and 1969, Medicare costs rose around 40 percent each year, leading to Medicare acquiring a reputation both in Congress and in the administrative branch as a program with a potential to be an uncontrollable burden on the federal budget.

One clear result of the first two years of experience was that the rise in medical costs initially led to increased interest in national health insurance. For example, in 1968, the organized labor-supported Committee for National Health Insurance was created, and the American Hospital Association announced that it planned to study the feasibility of a national health insurance plan. Some of this push related to the experience in certain states with the Medicaid program for people who were poor, begun in the same time frame as Medicare. In the large states of New York and California, the Medicaid program brought about great financial pressures, as both much higher utilization than predicted and price increases made the cost of the program, both to the states and the federal government, much higher than expected.

Medicare turned out to be a more complex program administratively and in terms of controlling costs than Social Security. With Social Security, most administrative issues were internal. Moreover, pension expenditures were quite predictable and based on clear formulas. In contrast, Medicare costs varied based on how much older adults used care, varied based on how much physicians and hospitals charged for the care, varied by changes in medical technology that made new procedures available, and were an additional and difficult to predict push on rising costs for the Medicare program. Moreover, administration of many aspects of the costs was controlled not by the government but by fiscal intermediaries. While these groups provided a buffer between the Social Security Administration and physicians and hospitals, they also weakened government control. The lack of clear definitions of terms and procedures left open the possibility that providers could increase their revenue in ways that the government had not anticipated. As the program was implemented, Social Security administrators, not yet that experienced with working with healthcare, ran into a number of unanticipated issues. Social Security administrators' initial emphasis was on cooperating with providers so that they would be able to participate and have a smooth beginning, as they had in the 1930s with Social Security. Looking back, it is easy to criticize some early decisions, but when the program was first enacted, the mandate was to provide services to older adults without significantly interfering with the traditional organization of American medicine.

The Medicaid program is more complex in its administrative structure, although it follows a more standard pattern in healthcare of joint federal-state programs with a matching component in terms of funding. Medicaid was started as a program of medical assistance to public welfare recipients, with any particular state participating voluntarily. Thus, from the beginning, there was variability in coverage and amounts of services funded across the states, as well as in participation. By 1970, all but one state, Arizona, participated in the program. But not all states included all possible components. States had the option of extending eligibility to people who were medically indigent and not on welfare who had a borderline poverty level of income but earned too much to be eligible for federally subsidized welfare.

Under Medicaid, all states were initially required to provide at least five basic services: inpatient hospital care, outpatient hospital services, other laboratory and x-ray services, skilled nursing home services, and physician services. A large number of optional services, such as optometric services, were available for states to consider as portions of the program. States could also opt to provide more essential mental health coverage, ambulance transportation, and dental care but were not required to do so by the federal government.

While issues of administration of each program became clearer over time, and a concern about costs became common, controlling costs was not as easy. In the Medicare program, the rate of hospital cost increases slowed from 20 percent in the first year; over the next five years, it averaged 14 percent (West 1971). Similarly, while the rate of growth in physician fees was the highest in 1966 (7.8 percent), the rate over the next five years remained quite high, at 6.8 percent. These rates of growth in the costs of Medicare meant that by 1970, administrators within the federal government and both Republican and Democratic politicians all agreed that the increase in costs of medical care was becoming a crisis. One reaction to this was to focus on overall reform of the healthcare system, not just changes in Medicare or Medicaid. A different reaction was to focus on changes and initiatives within Medicare. A key issue in Medicare policy became the discussion of different ways to control costs through regulatory approaches and financing reforms.

In 1972, Social Security amendments established professional standards review organizations (PSROs). These organizations were established to review the care received by federally funded patients as well as to encourage health maintenance organizations, review capital spending of hospitals, and allow for federal support of state experiments with prospective payment systems. In 1974, the Health Planning and Resource Development Act, Public Law 93641, created over 200 health systems agencies to oversee medical planning and resources use. As various political issues shifted in the 1970s, no major national health insurance reform was passed. The partial planning–based reforms were eventually judged to be ineffective, became sources of political concern, and were dismantled. With the benefit of hindsight, most policy analysts now agree that these partial reforms were inadequate measures for controlling rising healthcare costs and did little to impact the basic inflationary structure of medical care in the United States.

One other issue that became clear in the first few years of Medicare (and one reason for continued discussion of some type of national health insurance) was that while Medicare greatly improved older adults' access to healthcare, it did not solve all problems in terms of access to care. Medicare imposed various limitations on coverage, and beneficiaries were responsible for considerable amounts of deductibles and coinsurance, both for Part A (hospital costs) and for Part B (physician costs). Also, Medicare did not really provide coverage for what we now call long-term care, although at the time, many people discussed the longer-term costs of chronic illness. Home health and nursing home services were mostly restricted to short-term stays immediately following a hospital visit. At the time, this coverage was comparable to many private insurance packages, but it was much less than had initially been proposed as part of Truman's national health insurance provisions and less than some poor adults had received under Kerr-Mills. Those provisions became part of Medicaid and eventually became one of the ways in which the Medicaid program in most states now pays as much in long-term care for poor older adults as it does for care of children who are poor and their mothers, the groups thought of as the main recipients of the Medicaid program when it was passed. Actually, only a few changes in Medicare coverage occurred in the early years of the program. For example, in 1967, a 60-day reserve for hospitalization and a 50 percent coinsurance rate were added.

Amendments to the Medicare and Medicaid legislation began only a few years after initial passage, with many having either the goal of extending the program or the amount of services provided or the goal of modifying institutional eligibility requirements and reimbursement schedules. The 1967 amendments featured expanded coverage for durable medical equipment for use in the home, for podiatry services for nonroutine foot care, and for outpatient physical therapy under Part B of Medicare, as well as an additional lifetime reserve of 60 days of coverage for inpatient hospital care over and above the 90 days of original coverage for any spell of illness. Certain payment rules were also modified in favor of providers.

Unsettled Times in Healthcare and Proposed Health Reform, 1969–1979

Significant changes to Medicare and Medicaid were incorporated into the 1972 amendments. Some new services, such as chiropractic services, family planning services, and speech pathology, were added. Persons who were eligible for cash benefits under the disability provisions of the Social Security Act for at least 24 months were made eligible for medical benefits under the Medicare program. Additionally, Medicare services were extended to people who required hemodialysis or renal transplants for chronic renal disease by declaring them disabled and eligible for Medicare coverage under Title XVIII. This aspect became known as the ESRD (end-stage renal disease) program. While this expansion represented a numerically small category of people eligible for Medicare coverage, the average medical expenses of those in the disability category was very high. At the time this provision was passed, some health policy experts believed this would be the model of expansion of Medicare as a form of universal health insurance—coverage to more and more people by adding various disease categories. However, the expense of the program and changing times and attitudes have resulted in no further expansions of Medicare based on specific disease categories. Moreover, growing costs would increase concerns about federal costs and overall costs in the area of healthcare in years following this 1972 legislation.

During the Nixon and Ford administrations, considerable conflict developed between the branches of government, especially between the executive and legislative branches, relating to domestic social policy. President Nixon coined the term "new federalism" to describe his efforts to move away from the categorical programs focus of the Johnson years toward general revenue sharing. In revenue sharing, federal dollars were transferred to state and local governments (often through block grants) for many different purposes with fewer restrictions, instead of the federal government specifying that funds should be spent on a certain type of program in the maternal and child health area or chronic disease control, for example. Congress had previously favored categorical grants with detailed provisions and control, while Nixon pushed revenue sharing and block grants to states. The Nixon administration, in contrast to Johnson's, preferred actions that involved the private rather than the public sector. Categorical programs continued to grow, but in healthcare, the huge growth of the Medicare and Medicaid programs swamped all other policy efforts. Health personnel policy throughout the 1970s shifted to focus more on areas with special needs, rather than on growth in all categories and places.

One of Nixon's second-term (beginning in 1972) goals was passage of more comprehensive national health insurance of some type. In fact, at the time, many health policy experts believed major legislation might be passed, as Democrats in Congress, led by Senator Edward Kennedy, from Massachusetts, were drafting such legislation and were in favor of it. A push from a Republican president made the passage of major reform appear possible, and both sides were interested in a compromise. However, during that term, the Watergate scandal grew in importance and overtook other legislative agendas. By the time Nixon resigned, the push for national health insurance had dissipated.

In any case, some important programs were enacted in the areas of health personnel and health facilities. Federal subsidies of hospitals and construction of other healthcare facilities were ended, partially as a reaction to skyrocketing healthcare costs. In their place, legislation such as the National Health Planning and Resources Development Act of 1974 inspired exploratory planning and regulatory mechanisms to control expansion of facilities. By the mid-1970s, health personnel policies began to focus on specialty and geographic misdistribution of physicians rather than physician shortages, and by the end of the 1970s, there was concern about physician oversupply. The 1972 amendments also were the first to help control the growing costs of the Medicare program. Among the most important of the 1972 modifications was the establishment of the Professional Standards Review Organizations (PSROs) to address problems of cost, quality case control, and medical necessity of services. Associations of physicians reviewed the professional activities of physicians and other practitioners within institutions. The use of PSROs by Medicaid was made optional in 1981; later federal funding for PSROs was deleted, but the initial goal of the program was to ensure quality of care and controlled costs. Another modification linked to cost control was the addition of a provision to limit payments for capital expenditures by hospitals that had been disapproved by state or local planning agencies, as a way to put some enforcement aspects into health planning mechanisms.

In 1976–1977, a major reorganization of the Department of Health, Education, and Welfare led to the establishment of a separate agency, HCFA (Healthcare Financing Administration), whose job was to assume primary responsibility for implementing the Medicare and Medicaid programs. This new agency took over functions that had been located in the Bureau of Health Insurance of the Social Security Administration (Medicare) and in the Medical Services Administration of the Social and Rehabilitative Services (Medicaid), and made issues of administration of Medicare and Medicaid more easily centralized but also more visible. A major set of amendments dealing with antifraud and abuse in both Medicare and Medicaid were passed in 1977. These strengthened criminal and other penalties for fraud, included federal money for state Medicaid fraud units, and required uniform reporting systems for participating healthcare institutions. These were attempts to control costs and ensure quality.

A specific set of cost control measures was passed in 1978 to deal with the ESRD program, the Medicare End-Stage Renal Disease Amendments. Incentives were added to encourage the use of home dialysis and renal transplantation. A larger variety of reimbursement options for renal dialysis facilities was also included. Studies of the diseases and their treatment were also allocated, especially those focusing upon possible cost reductions in care for the disease.

Few new policy initiatives in health occurred during the presidency of Jimmy Carter (1977–1980), due to both some lack of overall interest in the issue and failed attempts to have policies enacted such as new hospital cost containment. By the end of the Carter presidency, the climate for expansion in government programs was further diminished. By 1980, antiregulatory pro-competition approaches were gaining in popularity at the national level, as were pushes to give more autonomy and control to state and local units, rather than the centralized planning and regulatory programs that had been present in earlier decades. One major piece of legislation passed at the end of Carter's term was the 1980 Omnibus Budget Reconciliation Act or OBRA 1980. This act included extensive modifications in Medicare and Medicaid, with 57 separate sections. Many focused on controlling costs, although some also expanded services, continuing the tradition of contradictions within the legislation. For example, the home health services provision of the Medicare legislation removed the 100 visit per year limit but required that patients pay a deductible for home care visits under Part B of the program. The goal of these changes was encouraging home care over more expensive institutional care. Some new services and providers were added, such as alcohol detoxification under Part A of Medicare and nurse midwifery under Medicaid.

This focus on amendments to Medicare and Medicaid set the stage for the Reagan administration's efforts in health, many of which also focused on Medicare and Medicaid. The changes of the 1970s demonstrated the differing concerns of cost containment, rationalization of care, expansion of some services, and creation of new alternatives (such as the use of midwives for Medicaid that could be considered to have an expansion and improvement of quality of care goal along with a cost containment goal). They also demonstrated how these two programs increasingly became the focus of health-related legislation from 1980 forward. For example, coverage for some mental health services, services for people with disabilities, and alcohol detoxification exemplified how programs initially aimed at physical healthcare for older adults and care for some groups of the poor became a way to address growing health and societal problems. Expansions, however, are never without costs, and cost increases, overall concerns about the federal government's expanding role in the lives of citizens, and high taxes set the stage for a complicated period in health policy after Reagan was elected president in November 1980.

Limited Changes and Conservative Approaches: The Reagan-Bush Period, 1980–1992

In this time period, many important aspects of health changes and pushes for certain types of health reform were linked to the overall policy direction of first the Reagan administration and then the Bush administration that followed it. The phrase "the Reagan revolution" was used to refer to an ascendancy of conservative values and goals, which included questioning the role of government and a belief that the private sector was better able to accomplish many societal goals. While these notions were applied most strongly to economic policy, they also became part of discussions about how to deal with health problems at a philosophical level, if not a practical one.

Often, broader social and economic themes of an administration impact what happens in the healthcare sector, and those themes then may drive healthcare reform efforts. Reagan's administration began a significant reduction in federal spending for domestic social programs, including the elimination of revenue sharing funds that helped local areas have money available for health and other programs. Tax reduction for all became a major theme, and this led to significant increases in the national debt and consequently a decline in the capacity of the federal government to fund many domestic social programs. Connected to fewer funds being available was a goal of decentralization of program authority and of devolution of powers to the states as a broad philosophical approach. Block grants to states became one mechanism to accomplish this goal, and this approach was applied to many social programs, including health. Block grants gave states discretion in how funds were used and ended up increasing inequities between states. While the Reagan administration did not accomplish its complete goal of consolidating all 26 public health programs into two large block grants, it did succeed in combining 20 programs into four block grants, while 6 programs remained categorical.

Deregulation was one overall goal of the Reagan administration. This led to the end of federal health planning efforts, and planning-related legislation was not renewed in the 1980s. Given Reagan's political philosophy that government regulations should be reduced, funds for health planning were gradually eliminated. In fiscal year 1981, before Reagan was president, the entire health planning program was funded for $126.5 million. By fiscal year 1983, the funding level was reduced by 54 percent, and the president's budget had requested the removal of all planning funds. The Tax Equity and Fiscal Responsibility Act of 1982 (TEFRA) led to dropping requirements for local planning agencies known as health systems agencies (HSAs) and made optional the use of the quality control agencies known as PROs (professional review organizations) in hospitals that served patients funded by Medicare and Medicaid, whereas requirements for local planning agencies had previously been required (Kronenfeld 1997). From a philosophical perspective, the deregulatory attitude of the Reagan administration was grounded in a belief that regulatory costs exceeded the regulatory benefits (Williams and Torrens, 2008).

Consistent with the administration's philosophy, another reform reduced the role of the federal government in health personnel planning and training. Funds were drastically cut for new scholarships that had been provided through the National Health Service Corps to encourage physicians and nurses to work in underserved rural areas after their professional training was completed. Grants to health professional schools based on their enrollment (known as capitation grants) were either totally eliminated or drastically reduced. Student loan programs in the health professions were cut in half from fiscal year 1982 to fiscal year 1985.

Some of the reforms in healthcare appear partially contradictory. Funds were eliminated for health maintenance organizations (HMOs), despite the emphasis in the Reagan administration on a pro-competition model of healthcare. Under this model, HMOs as a mechanism for care delivery were part of increasing competition in healthcare, as multiple HMOs in the same geographic area would be able to compete for customers. The stance of the administration, however, was that federal funds were unnecessary to stimulate this competition, and private market forces should be sufficient to facilitate HMO growth.

Some legislative actions did not have major budgetary implications but rather focused on issues relating to quality of care. A last major piece of general health related legislation prior to the election of President Clinton was the OBRA 1990 (Omnibus Budget Reconciliation Act) legislation passed under Bush. This legislation included the Patient Self-Determination Act. Healthcare institutions participating in Medicare or Medicaid (i.e., virtually all medical care institutions) had to provide all patients with written information on policies regarding self-determination as to treatment and living wills. Additionally, facilities had to determine whether patients had advance medical directives. The goal for the legislation was to increase discussion and consideration about under what conditions a person might no longer wish to receive medical services. While institutions now comply with the legislation by having patients sign additional paperwork, it is not clear that the requirement has encouraged a real more sophisticated level of discussion about important end of life issues.

The majority of healthcare system reforms during this period related to Medicare and Medicaid, partially because these programs had become such a significant part of overall expenditures for healthcare. The Omnibus Budget and Reconciliation Act of 1981 (OBRA 1981) was massive in its impact and the number of changes to Medicare and Medicaid, with 46 different sections relating to the two programs. A number of things were deleted from coverage, including alcoholic detoxification facilities, and occupational therapy was no longer considered a basis for entitlement for home health services. The Part B deductible on Medicare was also increased. Matching federal Medicaid payments to the states were reduced by 3 percent in fiscal year 1982, 4 percent in fiscal year 1983, and 4.5 percent in fiscal year 1984, although the cutbacks could be lowered by 1 percent in each fiscal year if a state operated a qualified hospital cost review program, had an unemployment rate over 15 percent of the national average, and had an effective fraud and abuse recovery program. Prior to 1981, Medicaid required states to offer recipients freedom of choice in the selection of providers. After 1981, states could apply for waivers of the freedom of choice requirements and could require Medicaid recipients to receive care from a specially designated pool of providers, which was the beginning of mandatory Medicaid HMOs for some recipients.

The Tax Equity and Fiscal Responsibility Act (TEFRA) of 1982 made a number of important changes in Medicare and Medicaid. Copayments for basic services, previously prohibited by federal statute, were made optional for states under the 1982 Medicaid amendments. Regulations related to acceptable error rates for Medicaid were tightened. For Medicare, hospice services became covered. The most important changes were part of an effort to control rising costs. TEFRA set a limit on how much Medicare would reimburse hospitals on a per case basis and limited the annual rate of increase for Medicare's reasonable charges per hospital discharge.

Up to this point in the Reagan administration, many of the changes were fairly small and specific. Much larger overall changes in the reimbursement policies of Medicare were passed in 1983. The Medicare Prospective Payment system (PPS) was created, which based payments to hospitals on predetermined rates per discharge for diagnosis-related groups (DRGs) instead of the cost-based system of reimbursement that had in place since the initial passage of the Medicare program. In this 1983 act, Congress also directed the administration to study physician payment reform options.

The DRG payment system was a major break with how payment had occurred in the past and was a complex system that was regulatory in content. The federal government provided detailed regulations that explained how the new system would work and forced hospitals that received Medicare funds (basically all hospitals in the United States) to completely rethink their payment systems. For an administration committed to competition and the private marketplace as the determinant of the distribution of healthcare resources, this regulatory approach seems quite surprising. The Reagan administration, in this case, demonstrated that it viewed healthcare issues as less critical than many other policy areas. If rising costs in healthcare were going to make tax cuts and other policy goals of the Reagan administration impossible, then a regulatory strategy to hold down healthcare costs was important to enact, even if the approach was not philosophically consistent.

The DRG prospective hospital payment reform system did help contain the growth in hospital costs to some extent. Most hospitals in the United States are reimbursed by Medicare as part of this system, although psychiatric, rehabilitation, children's, and long-term care hospitals have a somewhat different arrangement. The rate of growth in annual hospital expenses did slow for a few years after the implementation of the DRG system, but then the rate of growth again began to increase. Some early fears related to the implementation of this system were that hospitals would discharge sick patients too quickly, which could lead to unnecessary readmissions. There was some evidence that this occurred during the early phases of the DRG payment system (Gay et al. 1989). Some reforms in payment for readmissions have occurred, so readmissions within too short a period of time no longer generate the start of a new DRG payment for that hospitalization. Overall, the system has led to shorter lengths of stays—about 0.9 days in 1984 and 0.6 days in 1985 compared to an average drop of 0.2 days per year from 1967 to 1983 (Koch 1988). It seems that most patients did lose access to care under the DRG reimbursement system (DesHarnais, Kobrinski, and Chesney 1987), and hospitals shifted more care into outpatient settings.

The DRG system did lead to a partial success in the containment of Medicare costs, as DRGs led first to a decline and then a stabilization in inpatient hospital use from 1987 to the early 1990s, while costs for outpatient hospital care continued to increase, as did costs for physician care. Overall, this meant that the total impact of the payment reform system on total costs was less than hoped. Many would agree that the DRG payment system has been a success in the United States, and this approach to payment has been adopted or discussed by a number of other countries, such as Australia, Belgium, Norway, Sweden, and Portugal. As with so many reforms that affect only one payer and one type of service, there is much room for hospitals and other providers to learn how to "game" the system, that is, to maximize revenue given the new rules. Many analysts contend that piecemeal reforms of the healthcare system generally lead to disappointing results after a few years.

In 1984, the Deficit Reduction Act (DEFRA) continued to make changes in both payments to hospitals and payments to physicians. Further amendments throughout the rest of the decade also made changes in both areas, and there were also other overall policy shifts. Looking first at hospital payment and general policy changes, the DEFRA legislation placed a specific limit on the rate of increase in the DRG payment rates in the following two years. The Graham-Rudman-Hollins Act of

1985 established mandatory deficit reduction targets for the five subsequent years. This significantly impacted Medicare, with cuts in payments to both hospitals and physicians. The Consolidated Omnibus Budget Reconciliation Act (COBRA) of 1985 adjusted payments under Medicare for hospitals that served a disproportionate share of poor patients. Hospice care was made a permanent part of the program. PPS payment rates were frozen for part of the year as a way to hold down health-care costs, and payment to hospitals for indirect costs of medical education were modified. More technical modifications continued from 1986 through 1989.

While many of the changes were attempts to control costs, some reform was directed at improving access to care and quality, even in the cost-conscious Reagan era. In the Medicaid program, expansion of services was included, with states being required to cover eligible children up to age six with an option for states to provide additional coverage up to age eight. Additionally, the distinction between skilled nursing facilities and intermediate care facilities was eliminated, and a number of features designed to enhance the quality of care in nursing homes were included.

The Medicare Catastrophic Coverage Act was passed in 1988 and might have led to a large expansion in Medicare benefits if it had not been repealed before it went into effect. This act included provisions to add coverage for outpatient prescription drugs, to add coverage for respite care, and to place a cap on older adults' out of pocket spending for copayments. The new benefits were to phase in over four years and be paid for by premiums charged to Medicare enrollees, including an income-related supplemental premium. This legislation was a major departure from previous policymaking in the area of social insurance because the expanded benefits were to be funded entirely by those who were current beneficiaries, and there would be redistribution of benefits across income groups as part of the income-related supplemental premium. Despite being supported at the time by President Reagan, majorities in both houses of Congress, and the nation's largest senior citizen interest group (the American Association of Retired Persons, or AARP), the legislation was repealed less than 18 months later after enormous criticism (Himmelfarb 1995). Wealthier older adults objected to paying the income tax surcharge and additional premiums. Many older adults with average incomes were upset to discover that what they considered the biggest need in the catastrophic coverage area, coverage for nursing homes and long-term care costs, was not included. Others failed to grasp what the extensions of the program would provide to them, even though the changes would have benefitted all older adults without supplemental coverage and might have provided those benefits at a lower cost to many of the people paying for that coverage. As is often the case in politics and public opinion, perceptions matter, sometimes more than facts. The pressure on Congress from both older constituents and interest groups increased, and the legislation was repealed before most provisions were implemented.

The other major area of reform within the Medicare program was to control physician costs, ultimately through a new physician payment approach. Some smaller changes were enacted first. In 1984, the Deficit Reduction Act (DEFRA) temporarily froze increases in physician payments under Medicare and mandated that the Office of Technology Assessment study alternative means of paying for physician services as a way to guide reform of Medicare. The major reform in physician payment was in the OBRA 1989 legislation. The Healthcare Financing Administration (HCFA) was directed to begin implementing a resource-based relative value scale for reimbursing physicians (RBRVS) under the Medicare program with a four-year phase-in period. The new system began in January 1992.

Previously, physicians had been paid on the basis of what their charges were for various services. In studies prior to the development of the scales, how long it took physicians to perform various kinds of tasks was determined. Each service was assigned a relative weight based on three geographically adjusted values for work, practice costs, and malpractice premiums. Thus, new payment schemes were created related to time and other resources used. For the final application, a scale of relative weightings or relative values was formed as the basis of the new physician reimbursement system for Medicare patients (Hsiao et al. 1988; Hsiao 1989). Physician groups launched protests in June 1992 when the initial draft regulations were first released. The AMA (American Medical Association) was so upset that it threatened to seek congressional action to change the proposed system of reimbursement (McIlrath 1991a). Physicians argued that the reimbursement scheme was not fair and that transition rules were particularly inappropriate (McIlrath 1991b). Based on complaints in reaction to the initial drafts, HCFA did revise the rules somewhat. Whereas the initial regulations would have slightly increased fees paid to generalist physicians and decreased specialists' fees, negotiations with various groups from organized medicine, including the AMA, were used as a basis for some modifications.

One other reform included in the OBRA 1990 legislation aimed to simplify Medigap policies, which are policies older adults bought in this time period to supplement their Medicare coverage. Most of these policies covered some drug costs and the copayments that were required by Medicare. Before this legislation, Medicare beneficiaries had a choice of hundreds of Medigap policies, with widely varying benefits that were difficult to compare from one plan to the next. Because of the new legislation, by July 1992, all Medigap policies had to conform to one of 10 standardized packages developed by the National Association of Insurance Commissioners (NAIC). A study of the impact of this legislation showed that most consumers did learn to pick plans that better helped them with Medicare's cost-sharing requirements. Fewer consumers picked the more expensive plans that offered additional benefits such as preventive care, at-home recovery, or prescription drug coverage (Medigap Reforms 1996).

Medicare and Medicaid reform, especially related to payment of hospitals and physicians, yielded mixed results as viewed from a policy perspective. Although the elimination of regulatory approaches was one goal, this was accomplished only in the health planning area. Especially in Medicare and Medicaid, the Reagan and Bush administrations used regulations to limit hospital reimbursement and physician fees in the Medicare program. Even on a smaller scale, they used regulation to control the variety of Medigap policies offered to protect older consumers form purchasing worthless policies. Despite talk about stimulating pro-competition approaches, HMOs did not receive financial incentives, and growth in this area was modest in many sections of the country during this 12-year period. The largest impact on health services in this time period came from the dramatic reduction in federal fiscal capacity due to tax cuts, the growing federal deficit, and initial attempts to control the deficit. Congressional efforts focused on controlling cost increases through regulation rather than pro-competitive approaches. Even though the number of uninsured people increased in this 12-year period, access was not a major policy focus. Rather, most attention was given to controlling healthcare costs, partially because healthcare spending outpaced the growth of most of the economy. As often happens with a shift in political administration, the understanding of major problems in the health policy area also shifted gradually. The beginning of the Clinton administration arrived at a point of growing concern about access to care, costs, and attempts at large reforms.

Failed Attempts at Major Healthcare Reform in the Past Decades

Prior to President Clinton's first inauguration, there was discussion about the need for reform in the healthcare system. Most experts agree that if major reforms occur under a new president, they are most likely to succeed at the beginning of the term.

Not surprisingly, then, a push for major healthcare reform began to seriously take shape once Clinton was inaugurated at the beginning of 1993 and, in some ways, even earlier during the campaign. This push during the campaign included calls for changes in health insurance coverage within the United States, which were partially related to fears of unemployment, the overall economic climate, and its links to healthcare. This political interest in reform came from within the Democratic Party and those advising the presidential candidate that healthcare might be an important issue for winning an election. As the campaign developed, policy goals focused on picking a major domestic issue Clinton could affect, with the goal of gaining a second term and positively impacting the country.

Having good health insurance coverage has been one of the most basic indicators of access to healthcare services in the United States since the end of World War II. After the introduction of private insurance and its growth in the 1950s, issues of lack of health insurance coverage became a problem of special groups, such as older adults, the poor and more recently, the underinsured. Medicare helped deal with access problems for older adults, and Medicaid helped for some of the poorest people in the country. While estimates vary about the number of people who have been uninsured and underinsured in the United States since the early 1980s, most sources agree that the number of uninsured people rose from the late 1970s to the early 1990s (Access to Healthcare in the United States 1987; Andersen and Davidson 1996). In the late 1970s, the best estimates were that 25 to 26 million people in the United States were without health insurance (about 13 percent of the population under age 65). Estimates ranged from a low of 22 million to a high of 37 million by the late 1980s. In a review of statistics from 1980 to 1993, one source estimated that the uninsured population increased from 13 to 17 percent (Andersen and Davidson 1996). Medicaid coverage increased (from 6 to 10 percent) due to expansions in the program, but coverage by private health insurance decreased (from 79 to 71 percent).

The proportion covered by private health insurance decreased for every age group, and the decline was especially noticeable for children under age 15.

Critical to understanding the lack of health insurance in American society is the realization that most private health insurance in the United States is purchased through employer-based group insurance policies, which represent 75 to 85 percent of all private coverage. One major factor in the increase in the number of uninsured during the 1980s and early 1990s was the growth in unemployment in the early 1980s and again in the early 1990s.

People with a history of serious medical problems also often have no insurance. Many people with serious health problems do maintain health insurance coverage as long as they keep their jobs. If they lose their current jobs due to the general economy or their health but can still work, they may experience problems in finding employment due to their health. While people who are medically uninsurable are a small part of those without health insurance, they are important because they are very high utilizers of health services. In the early 1990s, it was estimated that 0.5 to 1 percent of the U.S. population was currently medically uninsurable.

In 1990, even with growing fears about lack of health insurance due to changes in the economy, both health policy experts and politicians considered it unlikely that there would be major governmental reform in healthcare (Skocpol 1995). However, some major pressures were building. The *Journal of the American Medical Association* published a special issue in 1991 focused on caring for the uninsured and underinsured. This resonated with the health policy community and physicians but did not lead to broad public discussion. Then, unexpectedly, in the summer of 1991, the type of event described by policy experts as a focusing event occurred (Kingdon 1984). Following the tragic death of Senator John Heinz in an aviation accident, relatively unknown (though he had been a long-time political activist) Harris Wofford became the Democratic senatorial candidate in a special election in

Pennsylvania. He aired a television commercial during the campaign that argued, "If every criminal in American has the right to a lawyer, then I think every working person should have the right to see a physician when they're ill." This spot resonated with the public and led his campaign to focus on calls for national health insurance. Wofford managed to defeat his opponent, and the Democratic Party began to realize that access to healthcare was an issue on the minds of the public.

During the Democratic primary debates, health insurance was a topic of major discussion. Several candidates developed well-reasoned, detailed proposals about health reform. While Clinton was not particularly identified with health issues in the early primary days, after being pushed by his rivals, he released a 10-page healthcare policy paper during the New Hampshire primary debates in January 1992. By the summer of 1992, when it was clear that Clinton had won the Democratic nomination for the presidency, he and his aides realized that healthcare could be an important issue in the upcoming election. In his acceptance speech at the Democratic convention at Madison Square Garden in 1992, Clinton vowed "to take on the healthcare profiteers and make healthcare affordable for every family." This rhetoric provided a sense of direction and commitment, but campaign advisors were leery of providing more details. Polls showed that voters wanted the system changed but were not certain what changes would help them (Johnson and Broder 1996).

After Clinton won the election in November 1992, the immediate issue was how important healthcare reform would become in his administration. For a politician who thought of himself as a policy wonk or detailed policy expert, was concerned about how presidents are viewed by history, and wanted to leave a lasting impact on the country, healthcare reform was the most challenging issue on the domestic agenda, and the one that would impact the greatest number of people. It was an issue about which everyone in the country shared some concern (which was in contrast to welfare reform, which would impact a more limited number of people). Five days after his inauguration, President Clinton announced the formation of the President's Task Force on National Health Reform. The job of the task force was to prepare healthcare reform legislation to be submitted to Congress within 100 days of the start of his term. Hilary Rodham Clinton, the president's wife, headed the task force. Despite expert advice against creating the commission, tackling overall healthcare reform as one big piece, and appointing his wife as the head of the commission, Clinton moved ahead with his plans.

Many of his aides at the time later argued that in some ways, Clinton's own intellectual capacities worked against successful healthcare reform. He was not intellectually inclined to follow advice that he should pursue more piecemeal reform efforts. He wanted a large impact, and he saw interconnections between health problems. He wanted to tackle the entire issue. A number of books and articles have reviewed in greater detail than is possible here how this effort at major healthcare reform faltered (see Starr 1994; Blendon et al. 1995; Johnson and Broder 1996; Yankelovich 1995). These analyses point out some of the difficulties with the commission, including problems with understanding the political process, weaknesses in overall Democratic strength and support of the plan, and problems in presenting the issue to the public. In addition, apart from the commission, there was a lack of significant interest groups to lobby for the plan, especially as groups opposed to the plan developed effective lobbying and public communication approaches.

Some experts argue that one important flaw in the process was the lack of a real public debate and public consensus over the issues (Yankelovich 1995; Blendon et al. 1995). Daniel Yankelovich, a public opinion expert, has argued that both the defeat of the catastrophic coverage plan for older adults in 1989 and the defeat of Clinton's reform plan in 1994 reflected a "massive failure of public deliberation" (Yankelovich 1995, p. 8). He argued that the nation's leadership class (including leaders of medicine, industry, education, law, science, religion, and journalism) did not talk effectively with the public. All the groups crafting the healthcare reform plan were from this leadership class, and the average American did not understand it. Because of this, Yankelovich argues that Clinton's plan lost public support, as its opponents found it easy to raise public fears about a plan people did not understand. In support of this argument, Yankelovich demonstrated that public knowledge about the plan decreased over time. Right after Clinton presented his health address to the nation, only 21 percent of the public said they knew much about it. By the next month, the numbers decreased to 17 percent and continued to fall until Congress considered the legislation in August 1994, when only 13 percent of Americans felt very well informed about the debate in general (Yankelovich 1995). If public support is to help push major reforms, the public must understand some aspects of the plan, at least enough to form an opinion about it.

If Yankelovich is correct that the defeat represented a massive failure of public deliberation linked to a lack of understanding about the plan, what did public opinion data show about overall support for the plan? Blendon and colleagues (1995) reviewed public opinion data and concluded that within a 12-month period, support for the plan fell from 71 to 43 percent. Although some of this loss was attributed to substantive choices, other reasons related to lack of communication with the public, especially the middle class, who became convinced the plan benefitted the poor more than themselves (which was perhaps part of the reason some Democratic politicians became convinced that they were going to lose the Senate over healthcare reform). In addition, the general public distrusted the government to do what is right most of the time, an important change from attitudes in the 1960s when Medicare and Medicaid were enacted.

The failure of Clinton's health reform effort was also partially due to process. A historian who reviewed the failure argued that the entire process allowed comprehensive healthcare reform to be defined too heavily as a purely presidential initiative and did not allow for either public involvement and discussion of trade-offs or for negotiations with Republicans who supported the general goal but did not want to contribute to the triumph of a new Democratic president (Heclo 1996). When compared to the success that President Johnson had in passing his War on Poverty legislation, including Medicare and Medicaid, President Clinton's reform came to be seen as a test of the president's personal popularity. A major difference is that Clinton did not have the large congressional majorities that allowed Johnson to successfully have legislation passed; nor did Clinton possess the understanding of congressional operations that Johnson had gained from his decades of service in the Senate and the strong personal contacts he had with senators based on that experience.

Not all process problems resulted from the Clintons' missteps. According to more recent reports, some conservative experts concluded that successful passage of a Clinton health plan would provide enormous trouble for the success of Republicans in the next sets of congressional and presidential elections. Bill Kristol, who worked for the conservative think tank The Project for the Republican Future, argued that congressional Republicans should work to kill, rather than amend, the Clinton plan as a way to enhance Republican chances of winning Congress and of becoming the majority party, a view that dovetailed with those of Newt Gingrich, whose Contract with America became a theme of the 1994 elections (Johnson and Broder 1996). Thus, Senate Republicans blocked the discussion of healthcare bills, as Gingrich did on the House side, and delayed any consideration of the health bill. The 1994 congressional elections had the potential to be significantly transformational. Republicans gained a majority in both houses of Congress, taking control of the House of Representatives for the first time in 40 years. Gains were large, with 52 seats gained in the House and 8 in the Senate. While healthcare was not the only explanation for why the Democrats did poorly in the election, the defeat of healthcare reform certainly played a role. One study (Blendon et al. 1995) examined public opinion survey data at the time of the election and national Election Day exit surveys. Most voters did not choose a candidate for Congress based on healthcare or even other national issues. Only 22 percent of voters said that candidates' stances on national issues were one of the most important factors, as contrasted with the candidate's experience, character and ethics, and political party. If voters were asked about concerns with specific issues, health became more important. Looking at data from Election Day surveys, healthcare was rated as number one in two of the surveys and tied for fourth in a third. Another question asked voters to name their top priorities for the new Congress. Only two surveys asked this question, and in both, healthcare was listed as number one. In examining issues of importance to voters and programs people support, voters were more in favor of providing health insurance to certain "deserving" groups. Voters favored covering children first and then other people who were uninsured. About half were willing to pay a modest increase in taxes or health insurance premiums to see some changes made in the healthcare system. Traditional Social Security and healthcare programs received wide support. Only 17 percent were willing to see cuts in Social Security or Medicaid as ways to deal with deficits, and even fewer (7 to 8 percent) were willing to see cuts in Medicare and veterans' benefits. There was much higher support for welfare cuts in programs such as food stamps, public housing, and AFDC (Aid to Families of Dependent Children).

The Republicans newly in control of both houses of Congress developed a plan to balance the budget by 2002, with large cuts (20 percent in Medicare and 30 percent in Medicaid). The budget passed but was opposed by Clinton. Government shutdowns occurred, first in mid-November and then again later in December, after a temporary spending bill expired. One major aspect of the budget disagreement involved cuts in Medicare and Medicaid along with other domestic programs. Eventually, the government reopened, and only modest cuts occurred in Medicare and Medicaid.

By the election year of 1996, everyone wanted a more successful session of Congress, and some minor health-related reforms were passed, such as consolidation of programs that provided primary healthcare centers in certain communities and some healthcare for the homeless. Two more important reforms were added related to mental health and HMO care, and the Health Insurance Portability and Accountability Act of 1996 was passed. This act had some important healthcare reforms. The mental health provision may be more important as a reminder of the importance of mental health than in any immediate changes made in the healthcare delivery system. It required annual and lifetime caps on mental health benefits to be at parity with those for physical illnesses. Some plans have had lifetime maximums of $50,000 for mental illnesses versus $1 million lifetime for physical illnesses. One limitation on the mental health provision is that it did not apply to small businesses with fewer than 50 employees.

The HMO provision was linked to maternity care and was a clear reaction to the growth of HMOs. To cut costs, some managed care companies put into effect policies that forced mothers to leave hospitals with their newborns fairly quickly, generally within 24 hours but in a few instances as soon as 10 hours after a normal vaginal birth. By the time the federal law was enacted, 30 states had already enacted provisions similar to the new federal ones that require HMOs to allow mothers to stay in the hospital up to 48 hours after a normal vaginal delivery and up to 96 hours after a Caesarean delivery. Thus, while the new law probably did not change the actual care available to many people, it sent an important message to HMOs.

The main portions of the Health Insurance Portability and Accountability Act involved helping people be less hesitant to take new jobs because concerns over loss of health insurance due to the reimposition of pre-existing clauses for serious health problems. The bill specifically prohibited employers who offered health coverage from limiting or denying coverage to individuals covered under a group health plan for more than 12 months if the individual had a medical condition that was diagnosed or treated in the previous 6 months. In addition, no new preexisting limit could ever be imposed on people who maintain coverage with no more than a 63-day gap, even if they change jobs or health plans. The legislation also prohibited employers from excluding an employee or dependent from coverage because their specific costs are too high. The legislation guaranteed renewability of health coverage to employers and individuals except in the case of fraud or misrepresentation. The legislation also provided for medical savings accounts as an option for small businesses and the self-employed.

SCHIP, Drug Coverage in Medicare, Medicare Managed Care Plans, and More Recent Changes in Medicare and Medicaid

In the fall of 1997, Congress passed the new joint federal-state Children's Health Insurance Program (SCHIP) as part of the Balanced Budget Act of 1997. This legislation was a major addition to the range of federally supported healthcare programs, Medicare for older adults, and Medicaid as a joint federal-state program for some poor people, and it began in fiscal year 1999. As an expansion, this program focused on providing coverage to children, as most people felt children should have access to health insurance. When SCHIP was passed, approximately 10 million U.S. children under the age of 18 (approximately 12 percent) did not have health insurance coverage. Children in some parts of the country and some population groups were more likely to be without health insurance, including children living in the South and the West, children living outside metropolitan areas, and Native American and Hispanic children, as well as the main target group of the legislation, children in lower income brackets. At the time the legislation was passed, children in the lowest income bracket were two to four times less likely than children in the highest income bracket to have medical insurance and a particular provider of care.

One of the misperceptions about Medicaid over the years has been that all poor children receive it. Traditionally, receipt of Medicaid was linked to receipt of other government subsidies (such as AFDC, Aid to Families with Dependent Children). The major changes in Medicaid in the 1980s extended benefits to pregnant women, infants, and children up to age six with family incomes below 133 percent of the federal poverty income guidelines. In 1998, regulations made it easier for states to extend Medicaid coverage to two-parent working families through the Section 1931 provision. Under this section, Medicaid eligibility was no longer tied to eligibility for welfare. Thus, states could no longer limit Medicaid only to children on welfare, and families have to actively enroll children in the program. Sometimes, eligible children are not enrolled. A study of Medicaid enrollment in 1995 concluded that about 30 percent of uninsured children nationally were eligible for Medicaid but not enrolled (Cassil 1997). The rest of the uninsured children were not Medicaid eligible. A different study (Selden et al. 1998) concluded that two out of every five uninsured children in the United States were eligible for but not enrolled in Medicaid. SCHIP aims to improve the rates of health insurance coverage among many of these children, including children of the working poor (which often includes parents who are in the labor force but work for an employer who does not provide healthcare insurance) as well as children from poorer families.

The largest expansion of health coverage since the passage of the Medicare and Medicaid Program was the SCHIP effort. For five years following fiscal year 1998, to help provide health insurance for children, $24 billion was made available. SCHIP has had some success in improving children's insurance levels. By 1999, public programs such as Medicaid and SCHIP covered 23 percent of children, compared with only

11 percent in 1987, before SCHIP and some Medicaid expansions (Federal Interagency Forum Focus 2001). The program provided states with much sought after flexibility in the ways in which they were allowed to expand coverage for uninsured children (Rosenbaum et al. 1998). Congress authorized up to $40 billion over 10 years after the success of the program was demonstrated in the initial five years. SCHIP is a federal grant-in-aid program that entitles states to elect to participate in federal allotments to targeted low-income children who are ineligible for other insurance coverage, including Medicaid (Rosenbaum et al. 1998). While the main purpose of SCHIP is to insure children not already covered by other programs (especially Medicaid or private insurance their parents receive as part of work benefits), a secondary purpose is to improve the quality of healthcare for the target population. However, no overall quality guidelines were developed. This left states to decide for themselves what "quality" healthcare meant. SCHIP is a federal means-tested public benefit and falls under some of the same immigration reform provisions as TANF (Temporary Assistance for Needy Families, the revised welfare program that replaced AFDC). This meant that states could not use funds to assist recently arrived (after August 22, 1996) qualified alien children (i.e., most noncitizen legal residents).

As the program became more fully integrated into child health policy and welfare programs, a crucial test of success became enrollment of children. Nationally, estimates were that only 75 percent of children eligible for Medicaid due to their family's welfare status were enrolled prior to the passage of the SCHIP legislation (Kids Care Tests 1997). Of children not receiving welfare who were eligible due to past program expansions, 45 percent were enrolled. Past experience with these programs demonstrated that if enrollment required complex forms and visits to local welfare offices, then many poor working parents (especially single parents who were more often women and minority parents for whom English was not their first language) did not enroll children. Initial experience with enrollment of children in SCHIP nationwide indicated that the program had mixed success. One estimate was that about 2 million children were enrolled by May 2000 (Friedrich 2000). Adding the experiences from the Medicaid program and from SCHIP, the percentage of low-income children covered by the programs increased from 29 to 33 percent initially, while the percentage of uninsured low-income parents increased from 31 to 35 percent (Friedrich 2000). Reports from a Robert Wood Johnson–funded study of the SCHIP effort were that many parents were not aware of the program, especially households with two working parents and with annual incomes above $25,000. Many of these parents did not realize their children could qualify for the program. In a special study of the design and implementation of the SCHIP program in six states (California, Colorado, Florida, Massachusetts, New York, and Washington), enrollment was found to be lower than initially expected (O'Brien et al. 2000). One possible reason was a more rapid decline in Medicaid enrollment than expected after the implementation of welfare reform. Systems intended to ensure that children of low-income families continued to receive either Medicaid or SCHIP (depending on total family income) even if the families were no longer eligible for welfare cash assistance (due to TANF time limitations and a return to work) broke down. Other issues were due to administrative and enrollment complexity, such as the difficulty of maintaining separate programs and being sure that families understood the different criteria. In some of the states in this study, language and immigration status were also barriers to enrollment. O'Brien and colleagues (2000) concluded that personal efforts to reach people would be required, along with greater education of low-income families about health insurance.

One enrollment limitation was a cost-sharing feature of the legislation. States could opt to include cost-sharing features either in the forms of premiums for the health insurance for families or copayments at the time services are received. Twenty-five states had such features; 12 used both premiums and copayments, 7 used only premiums, and the rest used a variety of more complicated processes (O'Brien et al. 2000). Premium payments provided both enrollment and logistical difficulties, especially because many poorer families live in a cash economy and have difficulty sending in monthly premium payments. Keeping up with the premiums was also difficult administratively, as the programs in many states had no experience with collecting fees from clients. Co-payments created fewer complications for state program administrators because such fees are collected not by the state agencies but by the providers of care at the time services are rendered. While families were supposed to be able to be reimbursed for these fees if they exceeded 5 percent of annual incomes, this requirement presented a major difficulty in maintenance of records.

In the early phases of the program, many states had difficulty reaching enrollment targets. In the initial year of operation, 36 states failed to reach their enrollment targets and thus had to return some of the federal money they had received, for example, Arizona had to return about $77 million in SCHIP funding, or about 66 percent of what had been received (Groppe and Chavez 2000). Arizona also provides an example of a state with special issues linked to large numbers of Latinos in the state. Although recent rulings by the INS (Immigration and Naturalization Services) have concluded that receipt of SCHIP funds will not count as a "public charge" and therefore will not hurt a family's chances of becoming eligible for citizenship, this concern has created an important barrier to enrollment in border states and others with large Latino populations. The stigma of a welfare program, the complexity of the application process, and the cost-sharing features were other barriers to enrollment in many states.

SCHIP has grown to be a major program, with expenditures totaling $2.1 billion in fiscal year 2000 (0.8 percent of total state healthcare spending and 0.2 percent of all state spending). By the next fiscal year, 2001, expenditures increased to $3.4 billion, representing 1.2 percent of total state healthcare spending and

0.4 percent of all state spending. Federal funds were a major part of the funding for SCHIP, and by fiscal year 2001, federal funds made up 69 percent of expenditures. This was higher than the proportion of Medicaid funding that came from federal sources, which in fiscal year 2001 was 56.5 percent.

By June 2003, SCHIP had become a major source of insurance coverage for children, with over 4 million children enrolled in the program, thus providing health insurance coverage to about 4 to 5 percent of all children. Though significant, this number was still much lower than the number of children in the Medicaid program. Between December 1998 and June 2003, SCHIP enrollment grew by about 3 million children. This rate of increase was much higher in the initial years of the program and then declined both due to program maturation and to cutbacks because of fiscal pressure (Kenny and Chang 2004).

This growth in numbers means that SCHIP has helped contribute to a decline in the number of children without health insurance. Numbers of uninsured children declined by 1.8 million between 1998 and 2002 (Kenny and Chang 2004). Given the program's focus on children from households with lower incomes, the reductions in the numbers of children without health insurance were particularly large for children who lived in households with incomes between 100 and 200 percent of the federal poverty level. In addition, many states reported higher Medicaid enrollment following the adoption of the SCHIP program, as parents applied for SCHIP but found their children were eligible for Medicaid. This helped decrease the number of children without health insurance.

Estimates are that since SCHIP was created in 1997, the number of uninsured low-income children in the United States has decreased by a third. In 2006, ninety-one percent of children who were covered by SCHIP had family incomes at or below 200 percent of the federal poverty level ($20,650 for a family of 4 in 2006). Combined with the Medicaid program that covers children in families with the lowest incomes,

SCHIP and Medicaid provide health insurance coverage to a quarter of all children in the United States and almost half of all low-income children.

Overall, SCHIP has been a very successful program, with states using federal SCHIP funds and some state funds to provide healthcare to children without health insurance whose families earn too much to qualify for Medicaid. There are important differences between SCHIP and Medicaid. Medicaid is a joint federal-state entitlement program. Federal funding increases automatically as healthcare costs and caseloads increase. In contrast, SCHIP is a block grant with a fixed annual funding level. The initial program was authorized for 10 years and must be reauthorized for higher funding levels to occur, and a debate over its reauthorization became one of the last health policy issues during the Bush administration.

Changes in Medicare, Especially Part D, Drug Plan and Managed Care Plans in Medicare, and Failed Reauthorization of SCHIP

Healthcare reform was not a major focus of the George W. Bush campaign, but some aspects of healthcare reform were discussed, especially a patients' rights bill, a variety of modifications in Medicare, and prescription drug coverage for Medicare recipients. The agency that administers Medicare and Medicaid received a name change, from the Healthcare Financing Administration to the Centers for Medicare and Medicaid Services (CMMS), and some expanded functions, but no major legislation was passed. In the summer of 2001, many experts expected some action during the next congressional session on those issues so that the Republicans would be able to point to some policy successes during the 2002 elections in November of that year. Instead, the terrorist attacks of September 11, 2001, occurred. Little domestic legislation passed in 2002, and the administration's focus was on foreign policy concerns, terrorism, and the declining economy that was partially a result of the attacks and partially due to scandals in the business community.

The presence of a Republican majority in the Senate, with a new Republican leader, Senator Bill Frist, who is a physician, helped focus some attention on healthcare issues in the second half of 2003. While there was growing concern about the rising costs of health insurance, the major health-related effort was a push for the passage of a Medicare reform bill. Both Democrats and Republicans wanted to return to their home states and be able to claim success in improving Medicare.

The Medicare Prescription Drug, Improvement, and Modernization Act of 2003 (MMA) was passed by the House (220–215) and the Senate (54–44) in November and signed into law (Public Law 108-173) by President Bush in December. This law provided a new outpatient prescription drug benefit under Medicare beginning in 2006. In the interim, it created a temporary prescription drug discount card and transitional assistance program. The temporary Medicare-Approved Drug Discount Card Program began in 2004; another transitional program provided a $600 annual credit to low-income Medicare beneficiaries without prescription drug coverage in 2004 and 2005. These programs were very confusing to older adults, although they were beneficial to some people.

In addition to the major drug benefit aspect of this bill, the MMA also made other important changes in Medicare. These included establishing a new income-related Part B premium for beneficiaries with higher incomes (beginning in 2007), indexing the Part B deductible so that it increases as the cost of living increases, and creating some changes to the Medicare HMO plans, known before this legislation as Medicare +Choice and now called the Medicare Advantage program.

The passage of the Part D Drug Option was a major addition to the Medicare program and dealt with what had been a major criticism of Medicare, the lack of drug coverage. Xu (2003), in an important article in *Health Affairs*, examined cross-sectional differences in the financial burden of prescription drug use among older adults in the United States and younger adult populations prior to passage of Part D. He used data from the 1998 Medical Expenditure Panel Survey to compare out of pocket spending for prescriptions, copayment rates, and the proportion of family income spent on prescription drugs for older adults versus working-age adults. Even after utilization or need was adjusted for, financial differences were still observed between older and younger adult populations. In particular, lower-income older adults were worse off than were younger adults in the same poverty class and their older peers in other income brackets.

Prior to the enactment of the Part D drug benefit, around a third of seniors had no drug coverage. People without drug coverage generally had higher out of pocket costs and were also less likely to fill prescriptions. Even a cost for a specific drug might be higher than that paid by younger people with drug coverage through an employer-based plan or retirees with certain drug coverage because some health insurance plans negotiate reduced fees for drugs for their plan members. However, Medicare beneficiaries without any drug coverage generally did not receive the discounts given to large insurers.

Medicare Part D is a prescription drug insurance plan that provides beneficiaries with prescription drug benefits. To receive these benefits, people must pay a monthly premium. People must choose among available plans in their state. The costs for the plans vary, as do the specific drugs that are covered. This can make the choice confusing to consumers, which was an initial concern as the program began. Because not every plan covers the same drugs, people must search the coverage options under the Medicare Part D plans available to them. Although consumers were confused initially, most are now choosing to enroll in a plan (unless they have supplemental coverage through a retirement work–based plan or other supplemental plan that provides comparable drug coverage). One other concern about the plan is that there is a coverage gap, or "donut hole." The donut hole aims to provide a large amount of coverage (75 percent) to most Medicare beneficiaries after the modest deductible but not be too expensive to maintain throughout the year. For those with extremely high drug costs (over $4,550 in 2010), catastrophic coverage resumes and covers the rest of their drug expenditures in that year. The donut hole has become one of the most controversial aspects of the Part D plan. The other controversial aspect is that the government is not allowed to negotiate drug prices, as it does on behalf of the Veterans' Administration and Medicaid.

After what most experts would describe as a difficult start, how well is Part D prescription coverage now working? This is an especially important question because this part of Medicare coverage is organized as a market in which consumers choose among different plans offered competitively by different insurance companies and health maintenance organizations. Nobel Prize–winning economist Daniel McFadden (2007) argues that after the initial confusion, people did participate in the program, with only 7.4 percent of the 65 and over eligible population not enrolling in Part D or a comparable prescription drug coverage plan. Average premiums, initially estimated to be around $37 a month, ended up lower than this. Because enrollment is voluntary, about 1.2 million seniors who use enough prescription drugs that they would benefit from coverage did not enroll, and these people tend to be more poorly educated and have incomes that put them above the poverty line. McFadden (2007) argues that consumers were fairly consistent in understanding their own self-interest and in selecting the lowest cost plan that provided good coverage given their health problems. He also stresses that one reason for this success was active management within Medicare, which worked hard to ensure that all plans were adequate and that consumers had ways to find out detailed information about the availability of drugs under different plans so that they could figure out which plans would work best for them.

Several articles published through the journal *Health Affairs* examined the effect of Medicare Part D coverage on drug use and cost sharing (Schneeweiss et al. 2009) and the effects of the coverage gap on drug spending in Medicare Part D (Zhang et al. 2009). Schneeweiss and colleagues found that use of some drugs such as statins and proton pump inhibiters stabilized at levels 11 to 37 percent above the trend in usage that would have been expected without participation in Part D of Medicare. For the 12 percent of people who reached the Part D coverage gap, there was a decrease in essential medication usage. Similarly, Zhang and colleagues found that those lacking coverage for drugs during the donut hole period reduced their drug use by 14 percent. The proportion of beneficiaries who reached the donut hole increased as their number of chronic conditions increased.

Another evaluation of the Part D drug benefit was conducted by Fisher and Rosenberg (2007). After reviewing some operational aspects of the program, which they argue began to improve as understanding of some of the details increased, they estimated an expenditure of $1,331 per beneficiary in insurance-covered drug expenditures, and a 10-year expenditure estimate of $520 billion, a figure comparable to Centers for Medicare and Medicaid Services projections of $534 billion. This projected figure by the Centers for Medicare and Medicaid Services is larger than the amount accepted by Congress when the bill was passed, which has led to concerns about the future of the drug benefit and Medicare, and the belief by Fisher and Rosenberg that cost reforms will be necessary in the future.

There have been critiques of this program. Many liberals believed the additional charges for Medicare for higher-income people might undermine the strength of the government's program and could be a first step in the dismantling of Medicare. Also, over time, middle-class older adults' commitment to the program might diminish if income ranges for the extra charges were not changed. The bill also provided substantial funding increases for some physician and hospital services but did nothing to control the costs of drugs. In the long run, some experts argued this could lead to even greater concerns about rising healthcare costs in future years.

The Medicare Prescription Drug, Improvement, and Modernization Act of 2003 (MMA) also modified the way that managed care plans worked in Medicare. In 1997, the Balanced Budget Act gave Medicare recipients the option of receiving their benefits through private managed care, then called Medicare+Choice plans, or through regular Medicare, which is the traditional fee-for-service program. That act authorized local preferred provider organizations (PPOs) as well as medical savings accounts and the establishment of a payment floor, which is mostly applicable to rural counties. Prior to this legislation, another version of Medicare HMOs was available in some locations as part of legislation that allowed private plans to contract with Medicare for reimbursement of costs related to providing care to Medicare beneficiaries. Today, the private managed care option is called Medicare Advantage, and it provides health plan options that are approved by Medicare but run by private companies. If a beneficiary chooses to participate in a Medicare Advantage plan, he or she will receive all Medicare-covered healthcare through the plan. Generally, this includes physician visits, hospital visits, and often prescription drug coverage. Some plans offer extra benefits such as coverage for vision, hearing, and dental issues not covered by regular Medicare. Often a person's out of pocket costs are less than what he or she would pay for regular Medicare without buying a supplemental Medicare policy.

The 1997 legislation that resulted in the Medicare+Choice plans was the result of the failure of some earlier attempts to modify Medicare and healthcare in general. After the failure of Clinton's healthcare reform 1993–1994 and Medicare's continued rising costs in the 1990s, the Republicans who controlled Congress in 1995 became interested in modifying Medicare's budgetary entitlement status. They were interested in a cap on health expenditures that eventually would convert the Medicare fee-for-service program into a defined contribution or voucher-type plan. As part of this effort, they wanted to have services to current Medicare beneficiaries be provided through private insurance plans. The Republicans hoped that this would increase enrollment of people over age 65 in managed care. It became clear to Republicans that the idea of taking away services currently available from the fee-for-service program was too unpopular politically, but the idea of weaning older adults from the original program into managed care options remained a goal, along with strict limits on spending overall. President Clinton and Democrats in Congress opposed these reforms. Although legislation was passed in 1995 with an almost exclusively partisan vote, President Clinton vetoed it. Party differences on Medicare became part of the 1996 presidential campaign in which Bill Clinton defeated Bob Dole.

By 1997, however, concerns about rising costs and interest in HMOs as a way to reform part of Medicare were still issues that resulted in the Balanced Budget Act of 1997. This act made a number of changes in Medicare, including encouraging HMO options, this time with bipartisan support. For Republicans and the managed care industry, the 1997 reforms were a beginning step toward the possibility of transforming Medicare into a competitive market. For Democrats, the reforms retained a commitment to the Medicare fee-for-service option in that beneficiaries would not be financially penalized for staying in the traditional Medicare option. In addition, both sides realized that deficit pressures in the program were real and that Medicare spending reductions would be important if there was a desire to have a balanced federal budget. Some health policy experts did view this change as the beginning of a change in Medicare from being in many ways a single-payer system to a health insurance market. At the time, managed care was becoming a dominant model across U.S. healthcare, and the new legislation extended that optimism about the benefits of managed care to those participants in the Medicare program who elected to participate in the HMO option. Early estimates from the Congressional Budget Office were that 27 percent of Medicare beneficiaries would pick the Medicare+Choice plans in 2002 and the number would grow to 35 percent by 2005 (Christensen 1998). These estimates were too high; only 11 percent of beneficiaries were in an HMO-type plan in 2004, and 22 percent of Medicare enrollees in 2009 picked a Medicare Advantage plan (Kaiser Family Foundation 2009).

There are some advantages to being enrolled in the Medicare Advantage plans. Participants do not need to purchase a supplemental Medigap policy and may have lower out of pocket costs, but in exchange, they have restricted choice in physicians and hospitals. A number of studies have compared Medicare fee-for-service and managed care plans, focusing on differences in quality of care. Medicare managed care plans overall did not appear to offer as high a quality of care. Referral rates, the rate of inpatient versus outpatient care, and length of hospital visits were all lower in managed care plans (Wong and Hellinger 2001). One study reported that managed care enrollees were less likely to receive needed coronary angiography, a potentially lifesaving procedure, after a heart attack (AHRQ 2000). Another study compared outcomes among chronically ill Medicare beneficiaries in fee-for-service and managed care plans (Ware et al. 1996) and found managed care enrollees experienced greater declines in physical health compared to fee-for-service enrollees. The same study also reported that those in poverty had better physical and mental health outcomes in fee-for-service plans, although those above poverty experienced better outcomes in managed care plans. Another aspect of quality of care is use of preventive care. Managed care Medicare plans look better by this measure, with studies showing increased attention to preventive care among some Medicare managed care plans, although there is much regional variation in the provision of preventive care by managed care plans (Moran 1999).

Hacker (2003) argued Medicare reform needs to be universal (i.e., for all Medicare enrollees), as opposed to only lodged within managed care. This option would be more costly overall for the government but would benefit all older adults equally, rich and poor, sick and healthy, in keeping with the program's original grounding as a social insurance plan. By 2003, a number of experts on Medicare such as Jonathan Oberlander (2003) were concluding that Medicare+Choice was a policy failure due to declining enrollment and an array of other problems already mentioned. Two recent discussions of the Medicare Advantage program tend to support the concern about whether private health insurance plans as part of Medicare Advantage are really better for beneficiaries or the overall heath and stability of Medicare. Berenson and Down (2009) concluded that ensuring stable plan choices and providing extra benefits in these plans ends up costing Medicare extra money. They believe that policymakers should focus on leveling the public-private playing field and deal with fiscal issues. Gold (2009) conducted a review of plans, using both quantitative program data and qualitative data from telephone interviews with 19 plan sponsors that enroll over 3.5 million people. From both data sources, she concluded that the Medicare Modernization Act has expanded choice and the role of the private sector but has added to Medicare's complexity and costs and has created potential inequities.

Changes will occur in this program as part of healthcare reform. Changes in the Medicare Advantage program were a topic of discussion in the Obama administration prior to the more detailed discussion of healthcare reform. There has already been a proposal to try to save $177 billion over 10 years through a new competitive bidding system for Medicare Advantage plans. In 2009, these private plans received an average 14 percent—or $12 billion—more than the government would pay if beneficiaries enrolled in those plans had remained in the traditional Medicare program. The Obama administration's initial plan would have gone beyond other proposals to cut payments to Medicare Advantage plans. Under the Obama administration's initial proposal, companies in a given geographic area would submit bids to cover Medicare beneficiaries, as they do now. But they would then be paid the average of their bids plus some additional money. Insurers submitting below-average bids would receive the average payment; they could use the difference between their bids and the average payment to provide additional benefits to enrollees. Companies with above-average bids would charge members a premium to make up the shortfall between the average payment and their bids (Jaffe 2009).

References

Access to Health Care in the United States: Results of a 1986 Survey. (1987). Special Report Number 2. Princeton, NJ: Robert Wood Johnson Foundation.

Agency for Healthcare Research and Quality (AHRQ). (2000). *Coronary Angiography Is Underused for Both Medicare Managed Care and Fee-for-Service Heart Attack Patients.* http://www.ahrq.gov/research/nov00/1100RA1.htm.

Andersen, Ronald M., and Pamela L. Davidson. (1996). "Measuring Access and Trends." In *Changing the U.S. Health Care Delivery System,* edited by Ronald M. Andersen, Thomas H. Rice, and Gerald F. Kominski. San Francisco: Jossey-Bass.

Berenson, Robert A., and Bryan E. Dowd. (2009). "Medicare Advantage Plans at a Crossroads: Yet Again." *Health Affairs* 28(1):w29–w40.

Blendon, Robert J., Mollyann Brodie, and John Benson. (1995). "What Happened to Americans' Support for the Clinton Health Plan?" *Health Affairs* 14:7–23.

Cassil, A. (1997, Dec. 5,). "Uninsured Patients Do Suffer, New Survey Reveals." *AHA News.* 33(48):3.

Christensen, Sandra. (1998). "Medicare+ Choice Provisions in the Balanced Budget Act of 1997." *Health Affairs.* 17:224–231.

DesHarnais, Susan, E. Kobrinski, and John Chesney. (1987). "The Early Effects of the PPS on Inpatient Utilization and the Quality of Care." *Inquiry* 24:7–16,

Federal Interagency Forum on Focus on Child and Family Statistics. (2001). *America's Children: Key Indicators of National Well Being.* Washington, DC: U.S. Government Printing Office.

Fisher, Erin, and Margie Rosenberg. (2007). *Medicare Part D: An Evaluation of the Prescription Drug Benefit.* Center for Biology Education. http://cbe.wisc.edu/assets/docs/pdf/srp-bio/2007/Fisher.pdf.

Friedrich, M. J. (2000). "Medically Underserved Children Need More Than Insurance Card." *Journal of the American Medical Association* 283:3056–3057.

Gay, Greer, Jennie J. Kronenfeld, Sam Baker, and Roger Amidon. (1989). "An Appraisal of Organizational Response to Fiscally Constraining Regulation." *Journal of Health and Social Behavior* 30:41055.

Gold, Marsha. (2009). "Medicare's Private Plans: A Report Card on Medicare Advantage." *Health Affairs* 28(1):w41–w54.

Groppe, M., and A. Chavez. (2000, July 7). "Arizona May Lose $77 Million in Child Health Care Funds." *Scottsdale Tribune,* 1–2.

Hacker, J. (2003, July 2). "How Not to Fix Medicare [Op-Ed]." *New York Times,* 1–3.

Heclo, Hugh. (1996). "The Clinton Health Plan: Historical Perspectives." *Health Affairs* 14:86–98.

Himmelfarb, R. (1995). *Catastrophic Politics: The Rise and Fall of the Medicare Catastrophic Coverage Act of 1989.* University Park: Pennsylvania State University Press.

Hsiao, W. C., D. B. Yntema, P. Braun, and E. Becker. (1988). "Resource Based Relative Values: An Overview." *Journal of the American Medical Association* 260:2347–2353.

Hsiao, William C. (1989). "Objective Research and Physician Payment: A Response from Harvard." *Health Affairs* 8 (4):72–75.

Jaffe, S. (2009). *Competitive Bidding in Medicare Advantage.* Robert Wood Johnson Foundation. http://www.rwjf.org/ healthreform/product.jsp?id=43710

Johnson, Haynes, and David S. Broder. (1996). *The System: The American Way of Politics at the Breaking Point.* Boston: Little, Brown.

Kaiser Family Foundation. (2009, April). *Medicare Advantage Fact Sheet.* http:/www.kff.org/medicare/upload/2052-12 .pdf.

Kaiser Family Foundation, Kaiser Commission on Medicaid and the Uninsured. (2007, Jan.). *Health Coverage for Low-Income Children.* http://www.kff.org/uninsured/ upload/2144-05.pdf

Kenney, G., and D. L. Chang. (2004). "The State Children's Health Insurance Program: Successes, Shortcomings and Challenges." *Health Affairs.* 23:51–62.

"Kids Care Tests Whether States Can Handle Big-Time Responsibility." (1997, Nov. 10). *American Hospital Association News* 33:3.

Kingdon, John W. (1984). *Agendas, Alternatives and Public Policy.* Boston: Little, Brown.

Koch, Alma L. (1988). "Financing Health Services." In Stephen J. Williams and Paul R. Torrens (Eds.), *Introduction to Health Services.* New York: John Wiley, 335–370.

Kronenfeld, J. J. (1997). *The Changing Federal Role in US Healthcare Policy.* Westport, CT: Praeger.

Lee, Phillip and Benjamin, A. E. (1999). "Health Policy and the Politics of Health Care." In Stephen J. Williams and Paul R. Torrens (Eds.), *Introduction to Health Services.* Albany, NY: Delmar.

Marmor, Theodore R. (2000). *The Politics of Medicare,* 2nd ed. New York: Aldine de Gruyter.

McFadden, Daniel. (2007, Feb. 16). "An Evaluation of Medicare Part D." *Economist's Views.* http://www.typepad.com/services/trackback/6a00d83451b33869e200d8351a332c69e2.

McIlrath, Sharon. (1991a.). "RBRVS Launch Could Be Difficult." *American Medical News* 1:37.

McIlrath, Sharon. (1991b). "HCFA Issues Final RBRVS Rules." *American Medical News,* 1.

"Medigap Reforms Make It Easier for Customers to Know What They Are Buying." (1996, Nov.) *Health Care Financing and Organization News and Progress.* Washington, DC: Alpha Center, 4–5.

Moran, M. (1999, Feb. 1). *Managed Care's Unfulfilled Promise: Making Prevention Part of the Medical Culture Requires a Change of Values. Progress Is Coming, but Slowly.* Amednews.com. http://www.ama-assn.org/amednews/1999/pick_99/feat0201.htm.

Oberlander, Jonathan. (2003). *The Political Life of Medicare.* Chicago: University of Chicago Press.

O'Brien, Mary Jo, Meghan Archdeacon, Midge Barrett, Sarah Crow, Sarah Janicki, David Rousseau, and Claudia Williams. (2000). *State Experience with Access Issues under Children's Health Insurance Expansions.* New York: Commonwealth Fund, Publication No. 384.

Quadagno, Jill. (2005). *One Nation Uninsured: Why the U.S. Has No National Health Insurance.* New York: Oxford University Press.

Quadagno, Jill. (2004). "Why The United States Has No National Health Insurance: Stakeholder Mobilization against the Welfare State, 1945–1996." *Journal of Health and Social Behavior* 45(Extra Issue): 25–44.

Rosenbaum, Sara, Kay Johnson, Colleen Sonosky, Anne Markus, and Chris DeGraw. (1998). "The Children's Hour: The State Children's Health Insurance Program." *Health Affairs* 17:75–89.

Schneeweiss, Sebastian, Amanda R. Patrick, Alex Pedan, Laleh Varasteh, Raisa Levin, Nan Liu, and William H. Shrank. (2009, Feb.). "The Effect of Medicare Part D Coverage on Srug Use and Cost Sharing among Seniors without Prior Drug Benefits." *Health Affairs* 28(2):w305–316.

Selden, Thomas M., Jessica S. Banthin, and Joel W. Cohen. (1998). "Medicaid's Problem Children: Eligible but Not Enrolled." *Health Affairs* 17:192–200.

Skocpol, Theda. 1995. "The Rise and Resounding Demise of the Clinton Plan." *Health Affairs* 14:66–85.

Skopcol, Theda. (1992). *Protecting Soldiers and Mothers: The Political Origins of Social Policy in the United States.* Cambridge, MA: Harvard University Press.

Starr, Paul. (1994). *The Logic of Health Care Reform.* New York: Penguin.

Starr, Paul. (1982). *The Social Transformation of American Medicine.* New York: Basic Books.

Steinmo, S., and J. Watts. (1995). "It's the Institutions Stupid: Why Comprehensive National Health Insurance Always Fails in America." *Journal of Health Politics, Policy and Law* 20:329–372.

Strickland, Stephen. (1978). *Research and the Health of Americans: Improving the Public Policy Process.* Lexington, MA: Lexington Books.

Wallace, Helen, M. Gold Edwin, and Allen C. Oglesby. (1982). *Maternal and Child Health Practices: Problems, Resources and Methods of Delivery.* 2nd ed. New York: John Wiley and Sons.

Ware, J. E. Jr., M. S. Bayliss, W. H. Rogers, M. Kosinski, and A. R. Tarlov. (1996). "Differences in 4-Year Health Outcomes for Elderly and Poor, Chronically Ill Patients Treated in HMO and Fee-for-Service Systems: Results from the Medical Outcomes Study." *Journal of the American Medical Association* 276(13):1039–1047.

West, Howard. (1971, Dec.). "Five Years of Medicare: A Statistical Review." *Social Security Bulletin* 34:17–27.

Williams, Stephen J., and Paul R. Torrens. (2008). *Introduction to Health Services,* 7th ed. Clifton Park, NY: Thompson Delmar.

Wong, H., and O. F. Hellinger. (2001). "Conducting Research on the Medicare Market: The Need for Better Data and Methods." *Health Services Research* 36(1 Part 2):291–308.

Xu, K. Tom. (2003). "Financial Disparities in Prescription Drug Use between Elderly and Nonelderly Americans." *Health Affairs* 22(5):210–221.

Yankelovich, Daniel. (1995). "The Debate That Wasn't: The Public and the Clinton Plan." *Health Affairs* 14:7–23.

Zhang, Yuting, Julie Marie Donohue, Joseph P. Newhouse, and Judith R. Lave. (2009). "The Effects of the Coverage Gap on Drug Spending: A Closer Look at Medicare Part D." *Health Affairs* 28(2):w317–w325.

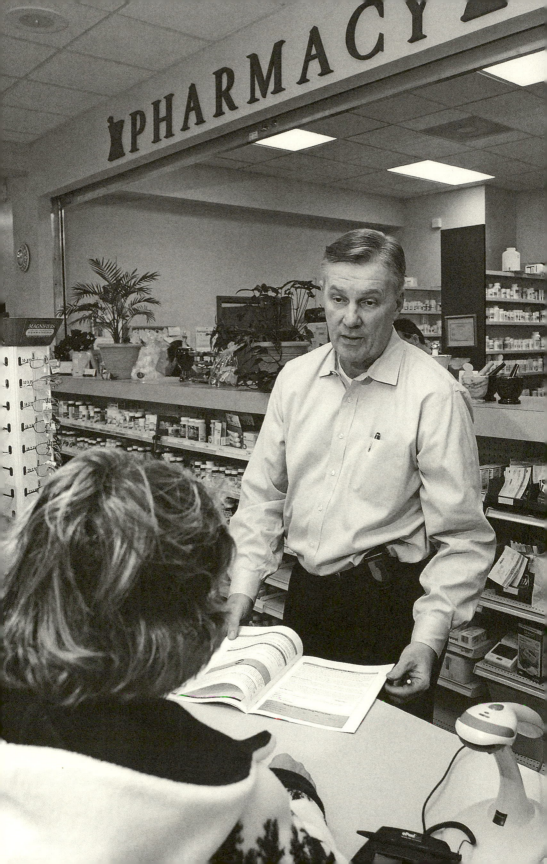

Introduction

The economic crisis of 2008 was the first and most important issue for the new Obama administration. While the economic crisis was of great importance, the costs and spending for healthcare were continuing to grow, reinforcing the need to look at healthcare reform. The amount the United States spent on healthcare continued to increase and is now at 17.6 percent of gross domestic product (GDP), roughly double the median share spent by the world's other economically advanced countries. Another way to think of this is that in 1970, $0.06 of every dollar spend in the United States was going to healthcare, but today it is almost $0.18 out of every dollar. Also, government programs for healthcare are consuming more federal spending. In 1970, (when Medicare and Medicaid had been in place for only five years), Medicare was 4 percent of federal spending, and Medicaid was 1 percent. By 2011, Medicare was consuming 16 percent of the federal budget, and Medicaid 8 percent. Costs have not gone up recently; rather, the cost of care increased over a number of decades.

Pharmacist Mark Doyle talks to customer Connie Whitehall, of Centre Hill, Pennsylvania, about her mother's prescription drug plan options on January 18, 2006. Following passage of Medicare "Part D" in 2006, pharmacists had to help customers deal with the complexities of the new drug benefit program. (AP Photo/Pat Little)

Since the 1970s, U.S. spending on healthcare has grown faster than the overall economy. Over the past 40 years, healthcare costs have grown more than 2 percent faster than the economy overall. Thus, once the Great Recession's immediate economic crisis related to banking was settled, it was important to address healthcare reform because healthcare was a growing and important part of the federal budget as well as an important issue for many voters.

Reauthorization of SCHIP in the Obama Administration and Other Smaller Reforms

One of the earliest pieces of legislation Obama signed once he became president, and his first health-related piece of legislation, was the reauthorization of the SCHIP program, on February 4, 2009. The bill reauthorized and expanded SCHIP to an additional 4 million children and was announced by President Obama as the first step to achieving universal health coverage in the United States. At the time, this legislation was explicitly viewed as a forerunner to major healthcare reform under Obama and a way to be sure that an important piece of health-related legislation that increased the number of children who had health insurance was continued.

The reauthorization of SCHIP legislation was really an unfinished piece of legislation left over from the Bush administration; without reauthorization, millions of children would have lost health insurance coverage. The legislation was originally set to expire on September 30, 2007, before the presidential election in November of 2008. Early attempts to reauthorize SCHIP were passed in August 2007, but with some important differences between the Senate and House versions. The combined version was not sent to the president. A compromise SCHIP bill, the Children's Health Insurance Program Reauthorization Act (CHIPRA) was passed in late September 2007. It passed 67–29 in the Senate. Of the 49 Senate Republicans, 18 voted in favor of the bill. In the House of

Representatives, the bill passed by a vote of 265–159. While this vote largely followed party lines, 45 Republicans voted in favor, and eight Democrats voted against. The bill would have resulted in a $35 billion increase over the following five years, bringing SCHIP's total costs estimated to $60 billion. To meet these higher costs, a $0.61 tax on each package of cigarettes sold was proposed. The first veto of this bill to reauthorize SCHIP occurred on October 3, 2007, after the objections from President Bush and Republicans in Congress that SCHIP was supposed to be a program for poor children, not middle-class children or adults. There was also discussion by Republicans that the tobacco tax increase being proposed was a regressive tax because smokers are more likely to come from lower income levels. On October 18, 2007, the House failed to override Bush's veto by a vote of 273–156, just 13 votes short of the two-thirds majority needed.

The second version of the bill passed the Senate with 64 positive votes and the House by a margin of 256 to 142. To try to meet some of the objections of President Bush (that it was too expensive and covered too many people), the second bill tightened restrictions against illegal immigrants, capped the income levels of families that would qualify for the program, and prevented adults from receiving benefits. But despite these modifications, this bill was also vetoed by President Bush. Eventually, through a continuing resolution that expired December 14, the legislation was extended at current fiscal year 2007 expenditure levels. After the results of the election were clear, President Bush signed an extension of SCHIP that did not include any expansion and lasted until March 2008, in time for the passage of new SCHIP legislation to be one of the first healthcare-related actions undertaken by the Obama administration.

Without congressional action, SCHIP was set to expire again on March 31. In the new legislation, children in families with incomes of up to three times the federal poverty level would qualify for the program. New Jersey and New York would be exempt from those income eligibility requirements and would be allowed to expand coverage to children in higher-income families. The legislation also required states to offer dental care through SCHIP and allowed them to extend dental benefits to children who had private coverage that did not include dental coverage. States were generally required to provide equal coverage for mental and physical illnesses under SCHIP. Another change in the new version of SCHIP was the elimination of a five-year waiting period for documented immigrant children and pregnant women to become eligible for the program. The measure required states to verify that SCHIP beneficiaries are documented immigrants or citizens, but this can be done by verifying eligibility through matching an applicant's name and Social Security number against federal records, rather than requiring documents proving citizenship. Under the legislation, SCHIP spending was increased by $32.8 billion over 4.5 years, and the increased spending was funded by a $0.62-per-pack increase in the federal cigarette tax. By 2013, the legislation provided coverage for an additional 4 million children, while continuing coverage for 7 million children already in the program.

Some other health-related pieces of legislation were also passed in Obama's first year as part of the American Recovery and Reinvestment Act (ARRA) of 2009. While this legislation, more popularly thought of as a stimulus package, mostly included regulations unrelated to health, a few important health provisions were included. One piece of the legislation paid for part of the cost of health insurance for people who lost their jobs involuntarily and continued their health insurance coverage through a COBRA plan (which allows people to continue their employer-based health insurance for some period of time after they leave or lose a job, if they pay for the complete cost of the coverage). The new legislation covered about 65 percent of the cost of the insurance through a tax credit provision. In addition, billions of dollars were made available to physicians and hospitals to help them implement electronic records as part of a push to improve the level of information technology within the healthcare system, with hopes that over a number of years, this would improve the efficiency of healthcare delivery. Beginning in 2011, the Centers for Medicare and Medicaid Services provided incentives to eligible healthcare providers who demonstrated meaningful use of certified electronic records, including making aspects of their medical records available to patients electronically.

Passage of Major Health Reform Legislation

The 2010 health reform legislation, now known as the Affordable Care Act (ACA), was the outcome of a push by the Obama administration to pass major healthcare reform legislation. The extension and expansion of the SCHIP effort was one positive move for the Obama administration, but the major focus on health for the first part of his term was a large, major health reform effort. From the very beginning, there were important differences of opinion within the administration about what major healthcare reform should include. There were also important political considerations. Most experts, and most of the political advisers within the administration, agreed that no matter what consensus might be achieved on what a "best" plan might include, it still might not be politically feasible. The politics of the process quickly became a major consideration, both in terms of what legislation might be more easily passed and what process would be used to pass legislation. For example, right after the election results were known, there was some discussion about whether it would be a good idea to use the reconciliation process to pass such legislation. This would require fewer votes, but it appeared that Obama and the Democratic Party might have the votes needed to pass more major health legislation without having to use the reconciliation process. When the formerly Republican senator from Pennsylvania Arlen Specter switched to the Democratic Party in April 2009, this increased the likely votes in favor of passage of some type of reform over the next 12 months.

Discussion about major healthcare reform had begun shortly after the election results were known. One of the Obama administration's initial approaches was to try and have

Congress work through and develop the legislation. Partially, this was a reaction to the failure of the Clinton plan, as the consensus of experts was that the Clinton administration had become too involved in the details, and Congress did not feel invested in the developing plan. So, the Obama administration's first goal was to ensure the program would eventually be enacted by involving congressional leaders and helping them have a sense of ownership over the process. Over the course of 2009, some criticism of this approach arose, concerning the president's involvement in major controversial legislation (Morone 2010). What clearly did happen was that at times, Democrats focused on congressional negotiations and in doing so, lost some control of the public debate. Right-wing populists, Tea Party activists, and other groups became part of a public debate filled with confusion and misrepresentation. As an example, a small provision that provided payment to physicians for discussing end of life issues with patients was publically debated on terms of "government death panels." During the summer of 2009, many older adults became panicked over this provision, and reforms began to lose some public support. When senators and representatives returned home for the summer recess, they held local discussions about the plan. In some states, these discussions became anything but calm, and both local and national media focused on congressional representatives and senators being shouted down at public meetings. Sometimes, the negative responses were organized by conservative groups; at other times, people reacted based on their own to fears and misinformation. By the fall of 2009, many congressional representatives and senators were convinced that portions of the bill that the public viewed negatively had to be modified. For example, the "death panels" debate resulted in the provision requiring pay to doctors for providing end of life counseling being struck from the Senate version of the bill.

In addition to providing Congress with a larger role in the creation of the bill, another lesson the Obama administration took from the Clinton defeat was the need to coopt potentially hostile industry groups. These groups were brought into the discussion early on, and deals were arranged with various groups to protect them against risks to their business in return for early support for healthcare reform (Miller 2010). Two important groups in this process were the pharmaceutical and hospital sectors. Each agreed to support some type of reform in exchange for negotiated limits on what they might lose. Each group was promised an expanded pool of millions of new customers, which would help make up for any losses from lower than desired reimbursement levels and new taxes on business operations.

Another initial part of this strategy was quick and steady progress in moving bills through Congress. The desired time line was bringing a bill to the floor of both the House and the Senate by July 2008. This did not happen. Later dates were set (August 8, later in the fall, and before Christmas 2009), and these deadlines were also missed. These issues were being discussed in the public media, and some of the sense of the inevitability of passage was lost. At the same time, there was still some feeling that Obama and the Democratic Party would have the votes available to pass major legislation because the conversion of the formerly Republican senator from Pennsylvania, Specter, to the Democratic Party had given the Democrats a veto-proof majority in the Senate.

Some deals had to be worked out with employer-sponsored health plans, especially as it became clear that such efforts were needed to reassure segments of the public already satisfied with their own healthcare that not much would change. This resulted in Obama's well-publicized comment that "if you like your healthcare plan, you can keep it." At some point, Democrats also realized that keeping funds from private insurance helped limit the government's costs of adding new people to the system.

While initially Republicans in Congress were seen as weaker as a result of 2008 election losses, as healthcare changes began to be discussed, Republicans realized that fears about healthcare rationing and expansion of a public plan option were generating concerns from the public that could be used to build opposition to the proposed plans. This allowed Republicans to develop a strategy of pushing to move more slowly and to find some political support among groups such as older adult voters who liked their Medicare plans as they were and feared that expansion of public programs such as Medicaid for the uninsured would come at the expense of benefits for older adults.

Throughout the summer of 2009, some aspects of the bill were repositioned and refocused. Instead of discussing healthcare reform, President Obama began to talk about health *insurance* reform, a less comprehensive approach. The initial goal of universal coverage for everyone became redefined as universal coverage for *almost* everyone, and some experts now believe that one measure of success for the programs after 2014 will be what proportion of U.S. citizens still remain without health insurance. Noncitizens, estimated at around 10 million, will not be covered. Also, by this point in time, any expectations of bipartisan compromise had disappeared, and earlier efforts to court Republican support stopped.

Modifications to major parts of the bills (the House and Senate version were somewhat different) to gain political support began with greater effort in the fall but focused more heavily on Democrats. For example, the final House bill that passed on November 7, 2009, involved a deal with right-to-life House Democrats that limited access to abortion services. The Senate version was not passed until Christmas Eve, 2009, setting the stage for difficult political decisions related to having any bill passed.

The Republican strategy of moving slowly was successful in some ways, and things did move more slowly than the Obama administration desired. One major change to the plans occurred at the time of the January 2010 special election for Ted Kennedy's Massachusetts senatorial seat, due to Kennedy's death in the summer of 2009. In a shocking result, a Republican captured the seat. In the media and among some members of Congress, this was interpreted as a negative vote for Obama's healthcare proposals. Some experts pointed out that Massachusetts was a state that already had a plan in place to ensure access to healthcare insurance for the majority of the public and that the change in party of the Senate seat was more likely due to specific issues in Massachusetts and some weaknesses of the Democratic candidate and the campaign she ran. Despite these comments, there was real damage politically in the changing sense of the difficulty of passing a reform plan. The loss of one Democratic seat meant the Democrats no longer had a veto-proof majority in the Senate. This meant that passage of the bill might not be possible without use of reconciliation. Some political experts even argued that reform was dead.

Major political discussions suddenly became imperative. At this point, President Obama became a very active participant with his Democratic colleagues, arguing that failure should not be an option. There was still reluctance to push the bill through the Senate under reconciliation rules. Another approach was to have House Democrats trust their Senate colleagues and pass the Senate bill intact, counting on later revisions. Eventually, House Democrats under Speaker Pelosi used this strategy. They approved the older Senate legislation verbatim and then passed a separate package of limited changes through the budget reconciliation process, under which only a majority vote of 51 votes in the Senate would be needed.

The initial Senate version of the bill was passed in late December 2009. The House of Representatives passed the Senate bill in March 2010 by a vote of 220–211. This bill to modify the Senate version also passed in March 2010. The bill was signed by President Obama on March 23, 2010, and is now known as the Patient Protection and Affordable Care Act of 2010.

The passage of any type of health insurance reform was a major political achievement for the Obama administration. Some experts argue that this was achieved by successfully

applying lessons learned from past failures, especially the importance of neutralizing interest group opposition (Oberlander
2010). Another important factor was a willingness to take some
smaller changes, rather than focusing on more comprehensive
changes. Despite the desire to have a public option included, it
was dropped when it appeared that it would doom the passage
of reform legislation (Halpin and Harbage 2010).

Coverage of the Legislation, Implementation Schedule, and Impact on Medicare

The Patient Protection and Affordable Care act of 2010, when
fully implemented, will help guarantee health insurance coverage for an estimated additional 32 million uninsured
Americans. Major coverage expansion began in 2014, with
exchanges being created and the requirement that most people
have health insurance, although a number of important provisions began sooner, and some provisions initially expected to
begin at an earlier date were delayed, such as the employer
mandate (see Table 2.1). Because of the renewal dates of many
healthcare policies, some changes, while implemented earlier,
were not felt by consumers until January 2011.

As of October 2010, insurers had to remove lifetime dollar
limits on policies, and some subsidies were available to small
businesses to provide coverage to employees. Insurance companies were barred from denying coverage to children with preexisting conditions. Children were allowed to stay on their
parents' insurance policies until their twenty-sixth birthday
(however, the issue of renewal dates meant that initially if a
child graduated from college in May 2010, the child might still
be without coverage for the rest of 2010). Some companies
agreed to help parents in this situation by allowing coverage
early, but many did not. States had to put into place a state-
based, high-risk pool program to offer health insurance to people with preexisting medical conditions who had been denied
coverage. This was a temporary program funded from July 1,

Table 2.1.   Original Implementation Schedule (and Some Modifications) for Aspects of Obama Health Insurance Reform Legislation

2010

- No Lifetime Limits on Coverage: started October 2010.
- State-Based Health Risk Pools: Establish a state-based, high-risk pool program to offer health insurance to people with preexisting medical conditions who have been denied coverage. Temporary program funded from July 1, 2010 through January 1, 2014.
- Protection from Cancellation of Existing Policies: Policies cannot be cancelled because of extensive claims, started October 2010.
- No Preexisting Exclusions for Children: Children cannot be excluded from a parent's plan for certain conditions, started October 2010.
- Extension of Coverage for Young Adults: Parental health plan is required to allow children to stay on family policy until age 26, started October 2010.
- New Prevention Benefits: New health plans must offer prevention and wellness benefits without out of pocket expenses such as deductibles and copayments for these services, started October 2010.
- Tax Credits for Small Businesses: Tax credit of up to 35 percent of the cost of health insurance premiums, started immediately.
- Medicare Changes: Rebate check of $250 if a beneficiary hits the donut hole in 2010, more funds to train primary care doctors, and an extra $11 billion over five years to expand community health centers.

2011

- Prevention and Wellness: grants to small employers to establish wellness programs for employees. Chain restaurants and vending machine companies must disclose nutritional content of each food item.
- Quality of Healthcare: New program to help community-based emergency departments and trauma centers. New programs to support school-based health centers and nurse-managed health clinics.
- Tax Changes: New annual fee for federal government from pharmaceutical companies. Changes in rules for health savings accounts to no longer allow over-the-counter medications. Higher tax on distributions from HSA that are not used for qualified medical expenses.
- Medicare: Annual checkup included at no cost to patient. If in donut hole, 50 percent discount on cost of brand-name drugs. No more cost-sharing for preventive services such as glaucoma tests, mammograms, and prostate cancer screening. Payment bonus of 10 percent to primary care physicians and general surgeons who practice in areas with a significant shortage of physicians, for 2011 through 2015.
- Long-Term Care: Start of CLASS Program, a national voluntary insurance program to provide individuals with a cash benefit if they have a functional limitation or disability.

(continued)

Table 2.1. (*continued*)

2012

- Medicare: Reduce payments to hospitals by a certain percentage if those hospitals have too many preventable hospital readmissions, as a quality measure. Create Medicare Independence at Home demonstration program to allow healthcare professionals to provide primary care services in the homes of Medicare beneficiaries at high need. Begin to establish a hospital "value-based" program to pay hospitals according to how well they perform on quality measures established by Medicare. Provide bonus payments to high-quality Medicare Advantage plans.
- Medicaid: Create demonstration programs to find more cost-effective ways of providing high-quality care. Some examples include bundle payment for episodes of care that include hospitalizations.

2013

- Health Insurance Reforms: Create Consumer Operated and Oriented Plan (CO-OP) program to provide loans and grants to create nonprofit, member-run health insurance companies.
- Quality of Care: Require the disclosure of financial relationships between physicians, hospitals, pharmacists, other providers, and companies that produce and distribute medications, medical devices, and medical supplies.
- Tax Changes: Threshold for itemized deduction for medical expenses increased from 7.5 percent of adjusted gross income to 10 percent of adjusted gross income. Increase in income-related taxes if a person earns more than $200,000 a year as an individual or $250,000 as a couple, including an extra charge of 0.9 percent for Medicare Part A; 3.8 percent Medicare tax on unearned income such as dividends and royalties.
- Medicare: In addition to 2012 change related to donut hole, begin phasing in an additional federal subsidy for brand-name prescription drugs (by 2020, this discount will be an additional 25 percent). Establish a national pilot program on bundled care similar to Medicaid change in 2012.
- Medicaid: Give funds to states to increase payments to primary care doctors.

2014

- Individual Insurance Coverage Mandates: All U.S. citizens and legal residents must have a "qualifying" health insurance, such as coverage through job, government plan (such as Medicaid, Medicare, Veterans' Administration, or being in the armed services), or a plan privately purchased; a tax penalty will be phased in starting in 2014 with a fine of $95 that will increase each year after that.
- Employer Insurance Mandates: Companies with more than 200 employees must provide employees with health plans, although employees may opt out of coverage; companies with over 50 employees without health insurance coverage will be fined $2,000 per full-time employee (penalties for employers delayed until 2015–2016).
- Health Insurance Exchanges: Beginning January 1, 2014, health insurance exchanges must be created, and an individual or small business (up to 100 employees) can compare the costs of various health plans and coverages as a way to make health insurance more affordable and easier to purchase for small

Table 2.1.   *(continued)*

businesses and individuals. The health plans must issue and renew policies without regard to any preexisting health conditions. Costs of premiums vary based on age, geographical location, family composition, and tobacco use. The yearly out of pocket costs are decreased based on income as a percentage of the federal poverty level. If family income is 133 percent to 400 percent of the federal poverty level, people may be eligible for a premium credit (or subsidy).

• Prevention and Wellness: Awards of 30 to 50 percent allowed for participation in wellness program and meeting certain health-related standards.

• Tax Changes: New annual fee required from health insurance companies.

• Medicare: Continue discounts for people in Part D coverage gap. Some changes to improve efficiency for Medicare Advantage plans. Establish Payment Advisory Board to submit recommendations to help reduce the growth in Medicare spending.

• Medicaid: Eligibility expands to include all Americans under age 65 with incomes up to 133 percent of the federal poverty level, including children, pregnant women, parents, and adults without dependent children. States receive additional Medicaid funds from the federal government to help pay for this. (Due to a U.S. Supreme Court ruling in 2012, the federal government is not allowed to take away funding from states that opt not to expand Medicaid, meaning states are not required to participate in the Medicaid expansions but may elect to do so.)

2015

• In October 2015, the match rate for states in the SCHIP (State Children's Health Insurance Program) will increase by 23 percent.

2016

• States will be allowed to form healthcare choice compacts; insurers can sell policies in any state participating in the compact.

2018

• Excise tax on insurers of employer-sponsored health plans with aggregate expenses that exceed $10,200 for individual coverage and $27,500 for family coverage.

2010, through January 1, 2014. As people began new health plan coverages at work or through private policies, those plans had to offer preventive services. In addition to parts of the legislation that impact individuals, there were provisions relating to improving the availability of healthcare, such as provisions to increase training of primary care physicians and more funds for community health centers.

In 2011, a preventive effort included grants to small employers to encourage wellness programs. Some tax changes began in 2011, with revisions to rules for health savings accounts so that over-the-counter medications would no longer be an allowable expense. A new program due to start, Community Living Assistance Services and Support (CLASS), was to be a national voluntary insurance program to provide individuals with a cash benefit if they had a functional limitation or disability, but this provision was deleted because it was determined by the Department of Health and Human Services that it was not financially sustainable (Emanuel 2014).

In 2012, Medicaid created demonstration programs to look for more cost-effective ways of providing care, such as using bundle payments for episodes of care that include hospitalizations rather than paying for each specific type of service that was received during that hospitalization.

In 2013, more tax changes became law, impacting the threshold for itemized deductions for medical expenses up to 10 percent of adjusted gross income. The Consumer Operated and Oriented Plan (CO-OP) program was created to provide loans and grants to exchanges and to other nonprofit member-run health insurance companies, and more rules related to providers of care were implemented. States received Medicaid funds to increase payments to primary care doctors.

The largest set of changes, especially for the typical consumer, started in 2014, when the individual insurance coverage mandates took effect. By then, individuals were required to have qualifying health insurance coverage through their work, Medicare, Medicaid, Veterans' Administration coverage, or a privately purchased plan. Those without coverage would face tax penalties. In addition to the individual mandates, companies with more than 200 employees had to provide health plans to their employees; smaller companies (more than 50 employees) had to provide coverage also, either through work or through the health insurance exchanges created by the legislation. (These employer mandates were modified and did not begin in 2014).

There were also some additional modifications to Medicare that began in 2014, such as continuing to deal with the prescription gap in Part D and the establishment of payment advisory boards, which some experts believe will be critical in trying to hold down rising costs of medical care overall. Medicaid initially was to be expanded to allow coverage for all Americans under the age of 65 with incomes up to 133 percent of the federal poverty level, with states receiving funds to help pay for this expansion. However, the U.S. Supreme Court ruled in 2012 that the federal government may not take away funding from states that opt not to expand Medicaid. Thus, Medicaid expansion was limited, meaning that states are not required to participate in the Medicaid expansions but may elect to do so. Taxes on high-cost health plans will not begin until 2017.

As is clear by the ways in which this legislation was gradually phased in, it is too early to assess the impact of the ACA legislation overall. Cutler (2010) argues that the true measure of healthcare reform's success will be whether it drives down medical costs over the long term. One of the ways the act is supposed to do this involves not how and whether individuals are enrolled in health insurance, but how medical services are bundled into larger payment groups, using values-based purchasing and improved coordination of care. The hope is that these changes will make the system more productive over a number of years. For the public, one important measure of success will be whether more people are able to obtain health insurance. Most experts agree that the reforms will create many new rules for all groups in healthcare, especially health insurance companies. The most significant changes will be in the small group and individual health insurance markets (Brennan and Studdert 2010). Some experts believe litigation and regulatory proceedings will determine the final shape of some of these new rules, making it difficult to make clear statements now about how some of the important features of the legislation will work after the first year of implementation. Some key decisions about how health insurance exchanges will work have been left to states, further complicating the issue (Kinsgdale and Bertko 2010).

The plans needed by states to implement the expansion of Medicaid for low-income adults became more complicated by a U.S. Supreme Court ruling in 2012 (Ku 2010). Not all states will participate in the Medicaid expansion. This could be a particularly difficult issue if current state budget shortfalls continue and the economic recovery is slow. Both as part of Medicaid and as part of Medicare, important administrative procedures include the establishment of a Center for Medicare and Medicaid Innovation within the Centers for Medicare and Medicaid Services (Guterman et al. 2010). How these new payment reform provisions are decided and implemented may be critical to the success of the new legislation. Because the legislation is new, and because so many important aspects are being implemented slowly and not explained in complete detail in the legislation, it will be important to observe the impact of this legislation as it is implemented. It is too soon to speculate on how well many of these detailed aspects of the plan will work.

Some of the changes in Medicare are among the more complicated changes to explain. Most Medicare recipients will continue to receive health insurance coverage through Medicare, not through the new healthcare exchanges. The ACA will reduce Medicare payments to the Medicare Advantage plans (the HMO option under Medicare). The legislation will make payments to Advantage plans equal (on average, per beneficiary) to payments through traditional Medicare. Until now, on average, Medicare Advantage plans received $135 more per beneficiary per month than the traditional fee-for-service Medicare plan. Although the bill will cut payments, no provisions cut mandated benefits. To deal with the reduction in payments, plans may cut extra optional benefits such as vision and dental coverage. Provisions for equalizing payments between Medicare Advantage plans and traditional Medicare are based on a recommendation by the nonpartisan Medicare Payment

Advisory Commission (MedPAC) and are supported by advocates for Medicare beneficiaries such as the Center for Medicare Advocacy. One purpose of these provisions is to extend the life of the Medicare Trust Fund, which, without some type of intervention, is projected to be depleted possibly as early as 2017. These provisions will result in approximately $118 billion in savings. There are some benefits for plans that perform well: a 2 percent bonus for plans that offer specified care coordination benefits and up to an additional 4 percent bonus if their quality is highly rated according to the Centers for Medicare and Medicaid Services (CMS) star-rating system.

One of the complicated areas of ACA relates to drug coverage under Medicare. Since Medicare Part D was enacted, there has been the so-called donut hole for some Medicare recipients. This coverage gap means that there is a temporary limit on what the drug plan will cover. Not all Medicare recipients enter the coverage gap, but for those who do, the coverage gap begins after the person and the drug plan have spent a certain amount for covered drugs. In 2014, once the person and the drug plan have spent $2,850 on covered drugs—at that point, the person enters the coverage gap. This amount may change each year—for 2015, the amount will be $2,960 for covered drugs. If a person enters the coverage gap, he or she will pay 47.5 percent of the plan's cost for covered brand-name prescription drugs in 2014 and 45 percent in 2015. For generic drugs, in 2014, Medicare will pay 28 percent of the price during the coverage gap. Individuals will pay the remaining 72 percent of the price. This amount will decrease each year until it reaches 25 percent in 2020. As part of passage of the ACA, Medicare recipients received a small rebate check if they hit the donut hole in Medicare coverage in 2010.

Other changes in Medicare included a 2012 drop of copays for annual checkups, glaucoma tests, mammograms, and prostate cancer screening. In 2013, the Independence at Home demonstration programs were created to allow healthcare professionals to provide some primary care services in the homes of Medicare beneficiaries; also, some changes were made in ways to pay hospitals and in the costs of Medicare Advantage plans. These latter changes are meant extend the life of the Medicare trust fund. As part of that effort, an independent advisory board was created to make recommendations for other cost savings.

Another complicated issue is how the healthcare exchanges and employer mandates will work. States can either create their own marketplaces or participate in the FFM (federally facilitated marketplace). In either case, the essence of how the ACA will keep the cost of healthcare down is premium subsidies. The subsidies include advance payment of tax credits for people with incomes between 100 and 400 percent of the federal poverty limit (FPL; $11,670–$46,680 for an individual in 2014) and cost-sharing reductions for people with incomes from 100 to 250 percent of the FPL ($11,670–$29,175 per year for an individual in 2014). In the initial regulations issued related to the ACA, the Internal Revenue Service (IRS) stated that the ACA allows premium subsidies for individuals who purchase coverage through both state-based marketplaces and the FFM.

The individual mandate portion of the legislation requires most Americans to have insurance or pay a tax. Some groups of people are exempt from the tax, including those whose annual insurance premiums would exceed 8 percent of household adjusted gross income. Other exempt groups are illegal immigrants, American Indians registered with a tribe, and people whose incomes are too low to have them to file federal income taxes. For most others, the premium subsidies will lower the cost of individual insurance.

Employers are also required to offer insurance, in a provision known as the employer mandate. Employers who do not offer insurance will pay a special tax called the employer shared responsibility payment. The employer shared responsibility payment will occur when one of an employer's full-time workers receives a marketplace premium subsidy. The employer mandate was delayed for the first year of operation of the exchanges in 2014 and will begin in 2015–2016. Small businesses with 50–99 full-time equivalent employees (FTE) will need to start insuring workers by 2016. Employers with 100 or more employees will need to start providing health benefits to at least 70 percent of their FTE by 2015 and to 95 percent of those employees by 2016. Healthcare tax credits have been retroactively available to small businesses with 25 or fewer FTE since 2010 to aid in the provision of health insurance.

Legal Challenges and Issues

Shortly after the legislation was signed, Florida and 20 other states filed a lawsuit challenging the constitutionality of the ACA, mostly focused on the individual mandate but also including Medicaid expansion and contraceptive coverage requirements. By November 2011, there were four federal circuit court rulings with different interpretations. Initial challenges resulted in differing decisions at regional-level courts; thus, the cases ended up at the U.S. Supreme Court.

In *National Federation of Independent Business (NFIB) v. Sebelius*, the Supreme Court upheld the constitutionality of the individual mandate but effectively made Medicaid expansion a state option. In terms of Medicaid expansion, access to Medicaid up to 138 percent of the FPL now depends on state of residence. While many states have decided to participate (28 as of 2014), others have not (23 as of 2014). This means that there are an estimated 4.5 million people with incomes too high to qualify for Medicaid but too low to qualify for marketplace subsidies in states that have not implemented the ACA's Medicaid expansion to date.

In *Hobby Lobby v. Burwell*, the Supreme Court ruled on a smaller issue but one of great concern to many women and their families that has received a great deal of public attention. In this case, the court decided that closely held for-profit corporations may exclude contraceptives from their health plan packages if their owners have religious objections. This issue is still partially under consideration because more lawsuits have been filed by nonprofit religiously affiliated employers challenging the ACA's contraceptive coverage requirement in the lower federal courts.

In addition, several cases challenging the availability of premium subsidies in the federally-facilitated marketplace (FFM) are currently progressing through the federal courts. All of this litigation has altered, or has the potential to alter, the way in which the ACA is implemented and consequently could affect achievement of the law's policy goals. In the current court cases challenging the IRS rule providing premium subsidies in the FFM, the ability of people to have access to affordable marketplace coverage also could depend on where people live. If the court rules against the ACA, state decisions to not expand Medicaid and also not create a state-based marketplace could have a compounded effect, with the result of even more people ending up with a more expansive coverage gap.

At the time of this writing, premium subsidies remain available in all marketplaces, and a final ruling on this issue is not expected for some time. In December 2014, the entire DC Circuit Court of Appeals will rehear the premium subsidy case. The court could uphold the current situation, reverse it, or modify the panel decision invalidating the IRS rule allowing subsidies in the FFM. Other similar cases are pending in federal district courts in Oklahoma and Indiana.

Enrollment Problems in Healthcare Exchanges

While the overall healthcare insurance reform efforts of the ACA are much broader than the healthcare exchanges, for the typical person, availability of the exchanges in January 2014 was viewed as the major rollout of the law. Thus, the creation of the Healthcare.gov website that was the route to the exchanges was very important in the public's image of how well the new law was working. Unfortunately, the beginnings of the website's operation were quite problematic, leading to many people being upset and tarnishing the image of the Obama administration and its hope for a successful rollout of the website and the exchanges. While the overall ACA includes much more than exchanges, and the exchanges include much more than the website, the fact that initially the website kept failing created a very negative image for much of the public. In retrospect, the federal government should have focused more on the creation of this complicated website. One issue was that while the people in charge of implementation were skilled in policy, they were not skilled in ecommerce or health insurance, or in managing such a complex website. The website was not well tested before being opened to the public, and major glitches quickly became apparent. With opposition to the ACA by conservative politicians and conservative media, the early computer issues allowed opponents to raise overall questions about the ACA and created prolonged negative publicity. In reviewing the experiences of some states that created their own exchanges, including a large state such as California, it is clear that private sector chief executive officers (CEOs) with many years of experience in working with private insurers *might* have created a better initial website. I emphasize *might* because not all states that created their own websites had positive initial experiences, including states such as Maryland, where the executive director was a former health insurance executive. In that state, the exchanges were such a mess that the director was fired near the end of 2013. A recent article reviewing the enrollment process concluded that although glitches and increased trouble-shooting are common when new information system technologies are introduced, the extent of technical difficulties both with the Healthcare.gov website and some of the state-based exchanges and websites was much greater than would be expected (Brooks 2014).

What were some of the things that went wrong, in addition to perhaps not having people with the right health insurance experience working on the websites? The negative political atmosphere was one factor. Another was that fewer states than expected decided to operate their own exchanges, meaning that to compensate, the workload of the federal government website ending up being larger than expected. Funding for the development of the website was inadequate, and the difficulties of the federal procurement process for computer technology made this worse, complicating the development of the product. The failures of the process were a combination of technical complexity, managerial challenges, and political challenges. Hindsight makes it clear that it might have been better to have delayed the start date and to give people more time to test the system before opening it to the public, but at the time, the political situation dictated pushing ahead and not publicly acknowledging problems. Even by the end of the initial enrollment period, some features such as account transfers to coordinate coverage with state Medicaid agencies and automation of the appeals procedure were not working well (Brooks 2014). The bad rollout, early technical glitches, and trouble with enrollment temporarily undermined public support for the ACA. However, the website was fixed, and expectations are that the fall 2014 enrollment should be much smoother. However, by November 2014, the website was ready to process renewals, and similar eligibility verification tools will need to be used and work better than they did in the initial enrollment period.

In addition to technical issues with the website, other enrollment-related problems were due more to the public not understanding the process. While the federal government spent money on outreach and public education for months before the website opened for enrollment, only a third of uninsured consumers understood that they could receive financial assistance to help with premium costs, and only one in five understood that there was a deadline to sign up for coverage to avoid a tax penalty (Brooks 2014). Most people said their most important source of information was the news, and the news sources were dominated by discussion of political concerns and website problems. In addition to issues with the website, call centers and navigators were supposed to be available to help, but as the website problems persisted, these sources were so overwhelmed that there were long phone waits. By the end of the enrollment period, these delays improved as the website did, but people who had tried to use the website or personal help in the early months of the enrollment period were discouraged.

There is hope for the future, as there may be a broader selection of health insurance plans in the future. Preliminary data from the government indicate that more insurance companies want to participate in the health exchanges for the 2015 enrollment year. This is true both for those states using the federal exchanges and for the 14 states that ran their own exchanges.

Early Evidence of Insurance Numbers and Costs of Healthcare

Before the ACA was passed, around 15 percent of Americans were uninsured. Many of those with insurance were covered through government programs such as Medicare and Medicaid, while others had private health insurance coverage, either through their workplace or purchased through the private marketplace as individual coverage plans. Even with all of the enrollment problems and problems with the exchanges, by the time enrollment had ended, around 7.1 million people had signed up under the ACA, close to the original goal of the Obama administration. The Congressional Budget Office estimates that this number will increase to 13 million enrolled by 2015 and 22 million in 2016 (Shear and Pear 2014).

In January–March 2014, the first three months the health exchanges under the ACA were in place, early numbers showed a 1.3 percentage point decline of Americans without health insurance, based on data from the National Health Interview Survey (Sanger-Katz, 2014). (Caveat: enrollment surged at the end of March and the beginning of April, which is after these initial government data were collected.) Later numbers that examined the data in more detail indicate greater improvement in coverage rates (Tavernise 2014). Using National Health Interview Survey data, the estimated number of uninsured Americans fell by about 8 percent in the first quarter of 2014 when compared with the same quarter in 2013. As expected, there was a greater improvement in states that elected to participate in Medicaid expansion. While these figures are encouraging, most experts point out that one cannot draw a firm conclusion from such early data and that past experiences with health insurance expansion programs (such as in Massachusetts) suggest that a three-year time period is really needed to gauge how well the program is working.

Some people who have had coverage for much of 2014 will lose coverage because they have not met certain criteria of the ACA legislation and regulations, such as proving they are U.S. citizens and submitting proof of income if a household is receiving subsidies. The estimate is that in October 2014, around 115,000 people will lose coverage because they were not able to prove they were either U.S. citizens or legal immigrants eligible for coverage under the ACA. In May 2014, almost 1 million people had discrepancies in their immigration and citizenship records. They were asked to send in supporting documents, and most did. Around 300,000 did not respond and were sent an additional letter, and 115,000 did not respond to this second request (Pear 2014). In addition to these problems, there are also households who have not correctly verified their incomes to be able to continue receiving subsidies for their health insurance coverage. While there were almost 1.2 million households with these problems, almost 500,000 have been resolved, and another 400,000 are working on resolution.

In contrast to some of these negative and more complicated issues, there is also some early evidence that the ACA is having a positive impact on healthcare costs, especially within the Medicare program. The Congressional Budget Office has reported that Medicare now in 2014 is spending $1,000 less per beneficiary than they projected four years ago. However, it is too soon to have a clear picture of overall costs, and this remains one of the questions to be examined in more detail once the ACA has been in place longer.

Future Trends and Unresolved Issues

While there are high hopes and some initial evidence that the new reforms in health insurance—a more accurate description than "healthcare reform"—will lower the rates of the uninsured, many problems still remain. The public option, a way to be sure that there is an affordable option for everyone, did not end up in the legislation, and while insurance companies must offer coverage to all people and there are healthcare exchanges, there is not a limit on what can be charged, so costs of health insurance are not as well controlled as many would desire. Going into the second year of the implementation of the exchange aspect of the ACA, there is concern that costs will increase, but it is too soon to know yet. Costs of insurance vary by state, so concerns about costs of insurance have differed. In addition, while the legislation does have some mechanisms in place to control healthcare and drugs' rising costs, experts suggested many more prior to the enactment of the legislation. Some experts fear that, as happened with the passage of Medicare and Medicaid in the 1960s, costs will increase, and the program will need additional reforms. One analysis of Congressional Budget Office projections on the cost of the plan concludes that it is built on a shaky foundation of omitted costs, premiums shifted from other entitlements, and questionable spending cuts and revenue increases (Holtz-Eakin and Ramlet 2010). However, Orszag and Emmanuel (2010) argue that this is not the case. Over the long haul, they predict the Obama healthcare bill will reduce rising healthcare costs and be an important factor in the control of these costs, especially through the tax on Cadillac health insurance plans (those plans with the highest coverage levels), spending to improve health technology, and establishment of the Independent Payment

Advisory Board (IPAB), which is tasked with devising changes to Medicare's payment system. Only time will tell how well these measures work.

Similarly, some people believe the ACA will lead to increasing numbers of employees deciding to opt out of employer-provided insurance, making the exchanges even more important and perhaps moving the United States closer to the model of single-payer health insurance that has been pushed for many years by many groups on the political left. However, at this time, it is much too early to know how employers will react in five to ten years.

How the new taxes and fines will work as mechanisms to ensure that all people purchase coverage remains to be seen as the different provisions of the Obama plan come into effect in future years. Orszag and Emmanuel (2010) argue that over the long haul, the Obama healthcare bill should be an important factor in the reduction and control of healthcare costs, but other experts disagree or believe that economic recovery may have more impact. The establishment of the IPAB, an independent panel of medical experts tasked with devising changes to Medicare's payment system, did not occur until 2014, and the tax on Cadillac health insurance plans does not begin until 2018, so whether the plan ends up helping control healthcare costs or becomes a source of rising costs will not be known for a number of years. Private health insurance companies have been raising the health insurance rates for people who obtain their health insurance via private individual policies, not through workplace policies. Another question is how much the costs of care under exchanges will increase in the plan's second year (2015).

Some issues related to Medicare have been dealt with (e.g., the donut hole in the drug plan), but the major issue of long-term care for older adults has not been. The CLASS act provision to deal in at least a limited way with long-term care issues was cut from the ACA. Past problems with the lack of long-term care coverage continue both for Medicare and for those covered by other insurance options (Kronenfeld 2011). Given the increase in the numbers of people who will need long-term care in the next 30 years (as the large baby boom generation comes to need long-term care), this remains an important area of healthcare that will need reform in the future.

Almost all health policy analysts agree that the Obama plan is just the beginning of major changes in how healthcare and health insurance work in the United States (Emanuel 2014). In that sense, healthcare reform is always a work in progress. New issues and concerns always arise that then become the next focus of public policy discussions and of proposed reforms for the future.

References

Aday, L., R. Anderson, and G. Fleming. (1980). *Health Care in the U.S.: Equitable for Whom?* London: Sage.

Aston, G. (1998, October 26). "Number of Uninsured Continues to Rise." *American Medical News*, 5–6.

Belcher, E. C. and M. R. Chassin. (2001). "Improving the Quality of Health Care: Who Will Lead?" *Health Affairs* 20:164–179.

Brennan, Troyen A., and David M. Studdert. (2010). "How Will Health Insurers Respond to New Rules under Health Reform?" *Health Affairs* 29:1147–1151.

Brook, R. H., K. N. Williams, and A. Davis-Avery. (1976). "Quality Assurance Today and Tomorrow: Forecast for the Future." *Annals of Internal Medicine* 85:809–817.

Brooks, Tricia A. (2014). "Open Enrollment, Take Two." *Health Affairs* 33:927–930.

Budrys, G. (2001). *Our Unsystematic Health Care System.* Lanham, MD: Rowman and Littlefield.

Cassil, A. (1997, Dec. 15). Uninsured Patients Do Suffer, New Survey Reveals. *AHA News* 33(48): 3.

Cowan, C. A., H. C. Lazenby, A. B. Martin, P. A. McDonnell, A. L. Sensenig, C. E. Smith, et al. (2001). National Health Care Expenditures, 1999. *Health Care Financing Review* 22:77–110.

Cutler, David. (2010). "Analysis and Comments How Health Care Reform Must Bend the Cost Curve." *Health Affairs* 29:1131–1135.

Donabedian, A. (1968). "Promoting Quality through Evaluating the Process of Patient Care." *Medical Care* 6:181–202.

Donabedian, A., J. R. Wheeler, and L. Wyszewianski. (1982). Quality, Cost and Health: An Integrative Model. *Medical Care* 20:975–992.

Eberhardt, M. S., D. D. Ingram, and D. M. Makuc. (2001). *Urban and Rural Health Charts: Health USA, 2001.* Hyattesville, MD: National Center for Health Statistics.

Emanuel, Ezekial J. (2014). *Reinventing American Health Care.* New York: Public Affairs.

Freeman, H. E., R. J. Blendon, L. H. Aiken, S. Sudman, C. F. Mullinix, and C. R. Corey. (1987). Americans Report on Their Access to Health Care. *Health Affairs* 6 (Spring):11–27.

Gardner, J. (2001, March 12). The 800 Pound Gorilla Returns. *Modern Healthcare* 31: 5, 15.

Greenberg, L. (2001). Overview; PPO Performance Management Agenda for the Future. *Medical Care Research and Review* 58:8–15.

Guterman, Stuart, Karen David, Kristoff Stremkis, and Heather Drake. (2010). "Innovation in Medicare and Medicaid Will Be Central to Health Reform's Success." *Health Affairs* 29:1188–1193.

Halpin, Helen A., and Peter Harbage. (2010). "The Origins and Demise of the Public Option." *Health Affairs* 29:1107–1124.

Harvard Medical Practice Study. (1990). *Patients, Doctors and Lawyers: Medical Injury, Malpractice Litigation, and Patient Compensation in New York.* Cambridge, MA: Harvard University Press.

Haywood, R. A. and T. P. Hoffler. (2001). "Estimating Hospital Deaths Due to Medical Errors." *Journal of the American Medical Association* 286:415–420.

Himmelstein, D. U., S. Woolhandler, I. Hellender, and S. M. Wolfe. (1999). "Quality of Care in Investor-Owned vs. Not-for-Profit HMOS." *Journal of the American Medical Association* 282:159–163.

Holtz-eakin, Douglas, and Michael J. Ramlet. (2010). "Analysis and Commentary: Health Care Reform Is Likely to Widen Federal Budget Deficits, Not Reduce Them." *Health Affairs* 29:1136–1141.

Institute of Medicine (IOM). (2001). *Crossing the Quality Chasm: A New Health System for the 21st Century.* Washington, DC: National Academy of Sciences.

Institute of Medicine (IOM). (1999). *To Err Is Human.* Washington, DC: National Academy of Sciences.

Kaiser Commission on Medicaid and the Uninsured. (2001). *Medicaid Coverage during a Time of Rising Unemployment.* www.kff.org/content/2001/4026/4026.pdf.

Kaiser Family Foundation. (2001). *Rising Unemployment and the Uninsured.* www.kff.org/content/2001/6011/6011.pdf.

Kingsdale, Jon, and John Bertke. (2010). "Insurance Exchanges under Health Reform: Six Design Issues for the States." *Health Affairs* 29:1158–1163.

Kleinman, L. C. (2001). "Conceptual and Technical Issues Regarding the Use of HEDIS and HEDIS-like Measures in Preferred Provider Organizations." *Medical Research and Review* 58:37–57.

Kronenfeld, J. J. (2011). *Medicare*. Santa Barbara, CA: Greenwood.

Kronenfeld, J. J. (1997). *The Changing Federal Role in U.S. Healthcare Policy*. Westport, CT: Praeger.

Kronenfeld, J. J., and M. L. Whicker. (1984). *U.S. National Health Policy: An Analysis of the Federal Role*. New York: Praeger.

Ku, Leighton. (2010). Ready, Set, Plan, Implement: Exiting the Expansion of Medicaid. *Health Affairs*. 29: 1173–1177.

Lazerby, H. C., and S. W. Letsch. (1990). "National Health Expenditures, 1989." *Health Care Financing Review* 12:1–26.

Lee, P., and A. E. Benjamin. (1999). "Health Policy and the Politics of Health Care." In Stephen J. Williams and Paul Torrens (Eds.), *Introduction to Health Services*. Albany, NY: Delmar.

Levit, K. R., S. W. Lazerby, C. A. Cowan, and S. W. Letsch. (1991). "National Health Care Expenditures, 1990." *Health Care Financing Review* 13:29–54.

Lohr, K., and S. A. Schroeder. (1990). "A Strategy for Quality Assurance in Medicare." *New England Journal of Medicine* 322:707–712.

Meckler, L. (2003, March 5). "30 percent in U.S. without Health Care Coverage in 2001–02." *Arizona Republic*, p. A17.

Miller, Thomas P. (2010). Analysis and Commentary Health Reform: Only a Cease Fire in a Political Hundred Years' War. *Health Affairs*. 29: 1101-11-5.

Morone, James. H. (2010). "Presidents and Health Reform: From Franklin D. Roosevelt to Barrack Obama." *Health Affairs* 29:1096–1100.

Moyer, M. E. (1989). "A Revised Look at the Number of Uninsured Americans." *Health Affairs* 8(Summer):102–110.

National Health Expenditures Tables. (2001). http://www.cms .gov/Research-Statistics-Data-and-Systems/Statistics-Trends

-and-Reports/NationalHealthExpendData/Downloads/
tables.pdf.

"National Journal Examines Rises in Health Care Costs."
(2001, June 21). *Kaiser Daily Health Policy Reports*. www
.Kaisernetwork.org.

Oberlander, Jonathan. (2010). "Long Time Coming: Why
Health Reform Finally Passed." *Health Affairs* 29:112–116.

Office of National Cost Estimates. (1990). "National
Health Expenditures, 1988." *Health Care Financing Review*
11:1–54.

Orszaj, Peter, and Ezekial J. Emanuel. (2010). "Health Care
Reform and Cost Control." *New England Journal of
Medicine* 363:601–603.

Pear, Robert. (2014, Sept. 16). "U.S. to End Coverage under
Health Care Law for Tens of Thousands." *New York Times*.
http://nyti.ms/1qXOzGi.

Prescription Drug Trends: A Chartbook Update. (2001). www
.kff.org/content/2001/3112. (Accessed 1 June 2001)

Robert Wood Johnson Foundation. (1987). *Access to Health
Care in the United States: Results of a 1986 Survey*.
Princeton, NJ.

Sanger-Katz, Margot. (2014, Sept 16.). "New Estimates on
Health Care Coverage Are Accurate but Outdated." *New
York Times*. http://nyti.ms/1uPYluD.

Schuster, M. A., E. A. McGlynn, and R. H. Brook. (1998).
"How Good Is the Quality of Health Care in the United
States?" *Milbank Quarterly* 76:517–563.

Shaneyfelt, T. M. (2001). "Building Bridges to Quality."
Journal of the American Medical Association 286:2600–2601.

Shear, Michael D., and Robert Pear. (2014, April 11). "Obama
Claims Victory in Push for Insurance." *New York Times*.
http://www.nytimes.com/2014/04/02/us/politics/obama
-to-report-on-progress-of-health-care-law.html?module

=Search&mabReward=relbias%3As%2C{%222%22
%3A%22RI%3A13%22}&_r=0.

Steinmo, S. and J. Watts. (1995). "It's the Institutions Stupid:
Why Comprehensive National Health Insurance Always
Fails in America." *Journal of Health Politics, Policy and Law*
20:329–372.

Tavernise, Sabrina. (2014, Sept. 16). "Number of Americans
without Health Insurance Falls, Survey Shows." *New York
Times.* http://nyti.ms/1sdGJ9b.

Thorpe, K, E., J. E. Siegel, and T. Dailey. (1989). "Including
the Poor." *Journal of the American Medical Association*
261:1003–1007.

Waldo, D. R., K. R. Levit, and H. Lazerby. (1986). "National
Health Expenditures, 1985." *Health Care Financing Review*
8:1–21.

Wilensky, G. R. (1987). "Viable Strategies for Dealing with the
Uninsured." *Health Affairs* 6:33–40.

Wilensky, G. R., and K. E. Ladenheim. (1987). "The
Uninsured." *Frontiers of Health Services Management* 4
(Winter):3–31.

Wilson, R. W., and E. L. White. (1977). "Changes in
Morbidity, Disability, and Utilization Differences between
the Poor and the Nonpoor." *Medical Care* 15:636–650.

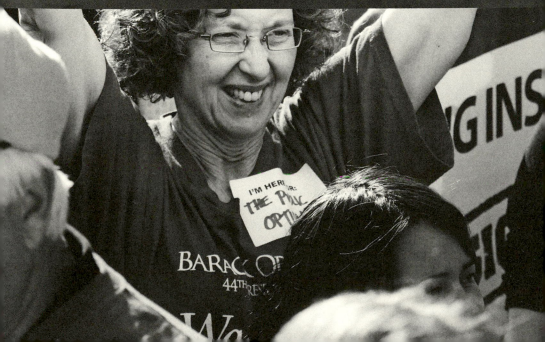

Introduction

This chapter presents essays from experts on specific aspects of health reform. They represent a wide range of viewpoints from liberal to conservative and from physicians to policy experts. The U.S. healthcare system is both vast and complex. These essays provide a feel for this complexity and the wide range of views on how to improve the delivery of healthcare in our country.

Healthcare Financing Reform in the United States: Leonard A. Cedars and Susan Cedars

The heated debate regarding healthcare financing and reform dates back to the earliest years of the twentieth century. One's attitudes toward healthcare reform are deeply rooted in how one views and defines healthcare. Some see equal access to high-quality healthcare as a basic right that should be afforded to those living in an industrialized country in the twenty-first century. Others view healthcare as a luxury, which should be available to those with the financial means of paying for it. For these individuals, marketplace factors dictate issues of

A demonstrator holds up a sign supporting a public healthcare option outside of a meeting of America's Health Insurance Plans on October 22, 2009. (Ryan Rodrick Beiler/Dreamstime.com)

access and quality. As was put to us recently by an acquaintance, "Healthcare is like a Mercedes. You only have a right to it if you can afford it." Our personal view of healthcare is that it is a basic right that should be equally available to everyone in the country.

The American people have been debating the merits of healthcare delivery models since around the time of the Great Depression. The most current healthcare reform law, the Patient Protection and Affordable Care Act (aka "Obamacare," or the ACA), was the result of growing intensity in this debate and intensified focus from an ailing healthcare industry. While the ACA was the most sweeping change to healthcare in our history, many are of the opinion that the reform did not go far enough to address the multitude of problems in the system.

Historically, health insurance in the United States has been provided for some, but not all, working Americans through employer-based health insurance plans. At the time of the drafting of the ACA, not all employers were obligated to provide health insurance for their workforce, and those that were, were not obligated to offer it to all employees. This left many working Americans without coverage. For them, the only avenue to health insurance coverage was to purchase an individual health plan at market prices. However, these market-based individual plans were not obligated to accept all applicants, leaving many vulnerable to rejection due to preexisting conditions; for many others who may have been eligible, costs were prohibitive. For retirees and the poor, Medicare, Medicaid, and the Children's Health Insurance Program (CHIP) were available. While this sounds like a multitude of options, the reality was that 46 million Americans were without coverage.

Some went without coverage by choice, hoping to maintain good health and avoid injury. When that strategy failed, they sought emergency care through hospital emergency departments and public or private charity clinics; many accumulated financially crippling bills for medical services. One of the greatest flaws in the pre-ACA system was that while there was no employer or individual mandate for coverage, hospitals, physicians, and other providers were mandated to provide emergency care. In summary, uncovered individuals were vulnerable to incurring unaffordable expenses, and providers were mandated to provide costly care, often with little or no hope for reimbursement.

In addition, the uninsured, whether by choice or by circumstance, tended to forego preventative care and often accessed the healthcare system in times of crisis, with advanced disease and in poorer condition, resulting in a much higher cost of care and a lower likelihood of good outcomes.

For the unemployed and truly indigent who received care from county clinics and hospitals, services often varied widely by locale and were difficult to access. Furthermore, this "safety-net" system was crisis oriented and often did not prioritize preventive care.

The purpose of the Affordable Care Act, as originally envisioned, was to bring about near universal health insurance coverage by:

1. Expanding the number of individuals covered under Medicaid programs to include all of the truly indigent
2. Mandating businesses to provide health insurance coverage for their employees
3. Mandating individuals to carry health insurance, either through an employer-provided health plan or through an individual plan purchased through the "healthcare marketplace"
4. Providing government subsidies, based on income, to help make the purchase of health insurance coverage more affordable for lower-income wage earners
5. Providing subsidies for small employers to help defray the cost of providing insurance to their employees

6. Making coverage available for purchase through insurance exchanges. One option available on the exchanges was to have been a "government option," that is, a government-administered healthcare plan that would compete with private insurers. The government option would ensure that the marketplace plans would be competitively priced

A variety of factors have hampered this legislation in achieving its goal of near-universal coverage:

1. As the bill made its way through the legislative process, the government option was dropped. A frequent criticism from many seeking coverage under the ACA is that they are finding rates higher than those they were previously paying. This may be an "unintended consequence" of the elimination of the government option, which would have provided an alternative to private insurers, who can set their rates at any level they deem profitable.

2. The expansion of Medicaid to cover more of the medically indigent population is dependent on individual states agreeing to participate in the expansion. Some states have refused to implement the Medicaid expansion, leaving a large number of individuals without coverage.

3. There has been almost uniform rejection of the law by the Republican Party. This lack of national consensus has fostered highly visible virulent opposition, portraying the new law as a negative draconian invention of the Obama administration: Obamacare. This campaign of misinformation, fear-mongering, and outright lies has left the public frightened, angry, and confused concerning the nature of the law and its potential benefits. As a result, many of those who would benefit most from the provisions of the ACA remain ignorant of its benefits and refuse to participate in the program.

4. Problems with the government website have hampered the public's ability to sign up for health insurance under the

new law and further increased their frustration and discomfort with the whole process.

5. A poorly orchestrated public education campaign has contributed to public confusion and frustration with the new law.

The ACA should have been welcomed by all Americans as a huge step forward in providing quality health insurance to all and greatly increasing access to care. The end result of the implementation of the ACA should be an improved level of health for the country, more efficient provision of healthcare, and less "cost-shifting" that results from providing uncompensated care to the uninsured when they present to hospital emergency departments in crisis.

While the law is not perfect in its current form, and would almost surely benefit from reinstatement of the government option, it is a good beginning in what should be an ongoing effort to improve access to affordable healthcare for all Americans. Hopefully, improved public education regarding the shortcomings of healthcare financing in this country and the potential benefits of the Affordable Care Act will overcome opposition from the insurance industry and other conservative stakeholders and allow our country to join the other industrialized countries in providing high-quality healthcare to all its citizens.

Leonard A. Cedars, MD, Maternal Fetal Medicine and Susan Cedars, Healthcare Executive

A European Perspective on the Affordable Care Act: Harry Perlstadt and Balázs Péter

From a European perspective, universal health insurance in the United States has been a long time coming. Almost all European countries have had either universal health insurance or a national health service since the 1950s. Europeans consider the health and well-being of individuals to be the responsibility of society. Europeans have higher social solidarity and are more concerned about the well-being of people from both socialist/communist political ideology and traditional Christianity.

In 1883 under chancellor Otto von Bismarck, Germany passed mandatory health insurance for indigent industrial workers and their families provided by nongovernment sickness funds with contributions from both workers and employers. By passing health insurance for some workers, Bismarck hoped to stymie his socialist opponents. Conservative governments followed suit and by the end of the nineteenth century, countries in the Austro-Hungarian Empire adopted this model. In Russia, the pre-revolutionary third duma dominated by gentry, landowners, and businessmen passed workers' health insurance in 1912. But in June 1918 after the revolution, the Bolsheviks established the People's Commissariat of Health to oversee all health work in Russia. In the United Kingdom, the Liberal Party under Lloyd George passed the National Insurance Act of 1911 with compulsory coverage for low-income workers, but not their dependents, with contributions from workers, employers, and the government. When the National Health Service was created in 1948, coverage became universal and comprehensive.

In 1891, Pope Leo XIII promulgated *Rerum Novarum*, in part addressing social insurance, which was perceived to be a threat to Christian charity work. The encyclical holds that governments should not intervene in matters that can be taken care of or resolved by families or communities and that public aid is acceptable only when a family cannot extricate itself from exceeding distress. It appears that Fascism more than Catholicism led to the introduction of compulsory health insurance in Spain, Portugal, and Italy in the 1930s and 1940s.

In contrast, more than many other peoples, Americans value individual freedom, autonomy, and self-sufficiency. Except in cases of national security (e.g., 9/11), Americans as a nation of immigrants have relatively lower social solidarity and are not strongly committed to the social well-being and development of all members of society. For example, in the late 1800s, many immigrant and religious groups built and supported hospitals so as not to be a burden on the larger society. Americans believe in controlling their own destiny and being responsible for their own well-being, including paying for their own health insurance. In addition, many U.S. ambulatory medical services, including physician offices and urgent care clinics, are considered to be businesses as compared with many hospitals, which are not-for-profit or government-run.

Almost all European countries provide healthcare insurance at the national level, publically funded through contributions or taxation, with some permitting private supplementary coverage paid for by employers or unions and/or individuals. Until the ACA, Medicare for older adults was the only nationwide public health insurance because Medicaid for the poor was controlled by each state. The ACA allowed the major private insurance companies such as Blue Cross, Aetna, and Humana to offer plans in each state that met the ACA coverage requirements.

European governments' health plans do not involve a complex system of premiums, copayments, and deductibles. The ACA does. For example, under an ACA platinum plan, the insurer pays 90 percent, and the plan member pays 10 percent out of pocket, while under a bronze plan, the insurer pays 60 percent and the plan member 40 percent. As a result, insurers charge a higher premium for a platinum plan than a bronze plan.

Europeans consider deductibles and copays to be a tool of consumers' cost-consciousness, and only the ailing part of the society is "punished" by paying copays, which are not of any concern to healthy people. The French health insurance system is the most generous, granting exemptions from coinsurance for treatment of 21 chronic illnesses and for people with invalid and work injury conditions. Children and low-income adults are also exempt from paying nonreimbursable copayments. Germany introduced cost-sharing for ambulatory care office visits to general practitioners, specialists, and dentists for adults in 2004 but dropped them in January 2013. Furthermore, the German type of social health insurance is based on the family principle so that a wage earner pays the same sum as a percentage of income regardless of marital status or number of dependent children. This percentage is lowered to 1 percent of annual gross income for qualifying chronically ill people who attended recommended counseling or screening procedures prior to becoming ill. In contrast, in the United States, a single person, couples without children, and couples with children pay different premium amounts, as do about the 10 percent of the German population who purchase private health insurance.

While many European countries have modified their national health insurance plans over the past 30 years, allowing some degree of privatization and local control, the political ideological battles over universal health insurance are over. But not so in the United States, where political ideology has been the focus of the passage and implementation of the ACA. Health is not a listed or defined right in the U.S. Constitution. Conservatives argue that health is a state or local responsibility, not one assigned to the federal government. It is, therefore, unconstitutional for the federal government to provide or regulate health insurance. Liberals argue that the preamble to the Constitution contains the phrase "to promote the general welfare," which has been used a justification for federal programs addressing national problems, including Social Security, health insurance for older adults (Medicare) and the poor (Medicaid), and environmental protection. They also argue that Article I, section 8, clause 3 grants Congress the power to regulate interstate commerce, which could include the sale of health insurance.

Yet almost from the beginning, the U.S. federal government has had a role in healthcare and health insurance. In 1798, Congress created the Marine Hospital Fund, which built and supported a set of hospitals in major ports to care for disabled and ill merchant seamen. It was funded by a tax of $0.20 per month from each seamen's wages that was collected at the port customs house operated by the Department of the Treasury. It was reorganized in 1871 as the Marine Hospital Service and became the Public Health Service in 1912. In 1879, Congress established a National Board of Health to collect information on public health matters and prepare a plan for coordinating quarantine regulations among the states to prevent the spread of communicable diseases such as yellow fever. But it was not reauthorized in 1883, partly because it conflicted with the health powers of individual states and municipalities.

The rise of the Tea Party and its subsequent role in the healthcare debate did not fit with the European model of multi-party coalitions. The Tea Party began in 2009 as a grassroots right-wing conservative protest movement against taxes and government intervention and spending in, among other areas, healthcare. It successfully supported some Republican candidates who were elected to Congress in 2010 and 2012. Despite being a minority in the House Republican caucus, it has been behind approximately 50 votes to repeal or defund the ACA.

In a European parliamentary system, a prolonged deadlock over an important issue such a healthcare would lead to a vote of no confidence, the prime minister resigning, and a new election being held. But U.S. congressional elections are held every two years, so notwithstanding Republican gains, President Obama was reelected to a second term in 2012, and the Democrats retained a majority in the U.S. Senate. However the U.S. House and U.S. Senate typically prepare different bills on the same topic. These different bills must then be reconciled, a single version must be passed by both, and this has to be signed by the president. This is complicated by a parliamentary rule in the Senate requiring 60 votes to close debate and call the question. This enables a minority to filibuster or otherwise block legislation it strongly opposes. Therefore, a super majority is needed in the Senate to pass or amend controversial legislation such as the ACA.

The Democrats had more than 60 votes for the passage of Medicare and Medicaid in 1965 but lacked 60 votes in the Senate when President Bill Clinton proposed his healthcare reform in 1993. They had exactly 60 votes for Senate passage of the ACA in late 2009 but lost it when a Republican won the late Senator Edward Kennedy's seat in a special election in early 2010. This made it difficult to make final adjustments with the House version and resulted in an ongoing stalemate. Therefore, President Obama has had to resort to executive orders to delay implementation of the employer mandate and the start-up of federal exchanges for small businesses, and to expand the individual mandate hardship waiver to those whose plans were canceled because they did not meet the ACA's minimum coverage requirements.

Unlike European conservatives a hundred years earlier who passed health insurance legislation in an attempt to take the issue away from liberals, American conservatives have steadfastly opposed any attempts by government to directly provide or mandate health insurance, and they thereby allowed liberals to enact legislation that is already benefiting many Americans and will be most difficult to completely undo.

Harry Perlstadt, PhD (University of Chicago), MPH (University of Michigan) is professor emeritus of Sociology at Michigan State University. His area of interest is medical sociology, and he has evaluated health programs for government and non-profit agencies. In 2010, he was a Fulbright lecturer on U.S. healthcare policy and politics at Semmelweis University, Budapest, Hungary. He is the recipient of the American Sociological Association's 2014 award for a distinguished career in sociological practice. Two recent publications are "Political Ideology, Party Identification and Perceptions of Health Disparities: An Exploratory Study of Cognitive and Moral Prejudice," in Jennie Jacobs Kronenfeld (Ed.), Research in the Sociology of Healthcare (Bingley, UK: Emerald Group, 2013) and "The Healthy Cities/Communities Movement: The Global Diffusion of Local Initiatives," in Jan Fritz and Jacques

Rheaume (Eds.), Clinical Sociology Perspectives *(New York: Springer, 2014).*

Dr. Balázs Péter is the vice director of the Public Health Institute at the Semmelweis University, Budapest, Hungary. The institute belongs to the Faculty of Medicine but has commitments also in dental and pharmaceutical training. The author started his career as a general surgeon in 1970 and has been working for 23 years in this specialization. Thus, he gained considerable knowledge about the day-to-day practice of out- and inpatient care. He started to research human resource problems of healthcare systems in the mid-1980s and has had an academic career only since 1994. Professionalism and medical business was the topic of his PhD theses. His main research areas are human resources of healthcare, especially workforce migration; historic roots and the present state of medical professionalism; the history of public health administration and of healthcare business; social health insurance; and health policy and system research.

Universal Health Coverage: The How and the Why: T. R. Reid

In the first decades of the twenty-first century, the United States is the richest, strongest, and most innovative nation on the planet. But in one key area of human endeavor—caring for the sick—the mighty USA is a third-rate power.

With tens of millions of people lacking health insurance, the world's richest country is the only advanced democracy that does not provide coverage for everybody. The Affordable Care Act (Obamacare) will help many Americans who were previously uninsured—but it does not get us to universal coverage. Even if Obamacare works precisely as it was designed, the Congressional Budget Office says, we will still have more than 30 million people uninsured in 2020.

Our country pays dearly, in lives and dollars, for this inadequate and inequitable system. The National Academy of Sciences says about 25,000 Americans die each year of treatable diseases for lack of treatment. Health outcomes in the United States lag behind results in other rich countries. One painful example is neonatal care. In the Commonwealth Fund's comparative studies, the United States ranks twenty-third out of the richest 23 countries in keeping newborns alive until their first birthday.

The crazy-quilt nature of our complex system is one of the major reasons we spend far more for healthcare than other advanced countries but get far less for the money. About one of every six dollars we spend pays for medical care or insurance. That's 17.5 percent of our total wealth—a far greater share than any other country spends.

But it doesn't have to be that way.

The United States could provide high-quality care to everybody at reasonable cost. I know this is true because all the other industrialized democracies have figured out how to do it. They provide coverage for all their citizens and all their resident aliens while spending, on average, about half of what we spend.

Which raises two pertinent questions: How do they do that? and Why do they do that?

How Do They Do It?

There are four basic models of healthcare systems around the world. Contrary to conventional American wisdom, these national models do not all involve "Socialized Medicine."

- The *Bismarck model,* named for its inventor, nineteenth-century German chancellor Otto von Bismarck, leaves healthcare to the private sector. In this system, everyone is required to buy health insurance from a private company; the doctors and hospitals are primarily private as well. Many Bismarck countries are less "socialized" than the United States. Germany, for example, has nothing like the U.S. Medicare system for older adults; Germans stay with private insurance cradle to grave.

- The insurers are private but subject to regulation. They have to pay every claim, generally within a few days. They can't use the "in-network" limitations common with U.S. insurance plans. In the Bismarck countries, you pick the doctor, you pick the hospital—and insurance has to pay. This private system of care is used, with some variation, in Germany, France, Switzerland, the Netherlands, Belgium, and Japan.

- In the *Beveridge model,* named for the British social reformer William Beveridge, healthcare is the government's responsibility, just like putting out fires or running the library. In this model, the government owns the hospitals and employs most or all of the doctors. There is no fee for any treatment. People have to pay, of course, but they pay through taxes, and then the government pays the doctor. This leads to high taxes—the sales tax in Britain is 20 percent on everything you buy. But with no insurance premiums or copays, people there end up paying much less than the average American.

- The Beveridge model is used in Britain, Spain, Italy, all of Scandinavia, and other countries. With the government providing and paying for the care, this system is probably what Americans have in mind when they talk about "Socialized Medicine."

- The *national health insurance model* is sometimes called the Douglas model, after its inventor, Tommy Douglas. Douglas was the premier (governor) of the Canadian province of Saskatchewan in the 1940s. At a time when roughly 15 percent of the population had health insurance, he created a system for 100 percent coverage, using a government insurance plan to pay private doctors and hospitals. This worked well, and by 1961, all of Canada had adopted it. The model has been adopted successfully in Australia, Taiwan, and South Korea. In Canada, the system is plagued by limited choice and long waits in some provinces, mainly because the Canadians have been stingy about funding it.

- Tommy Douglas came up with a catchy name for his government-run insurance plan: Medicare. In 1965, when the United States decided to provide health insurance for all older adults, we copied both the name Medicare and the model—government payment of private providers—from Canada.

These models of universal care are found only in rich countries. In most of the world, where healthcare is a luxury for the well-to-do, the standard system is called the *out of pocket model*. And it is exactly that. If your child is sick, and you have some money in your pocket to pay for care, she gets treated. If you cannot pay, the child stays sick or dies.

Why Do They Do It?

Why do most developed countries cover everybody? There are practical advantages. Obviously, healthcare for all saves lives; in Britain, Germany, Japan, and so on, nobody dies for lack of medical treatment. But it also saves money; all the countries with universal coverage spend far less than the United States—and that is not a coincidence. Covering everybody in a coherent system turns out to be cheaper than the fragmented, hugely complex contraption we are stuck with.

The main reason the world's rich countries provide healthcare for everyone, though, is a matter of morality. All the other industrialized democracies have committed to care for the least of their brethren—and especially for the sick. They see this as a moral imperative; frequently, religious beliefs underlie the design of the healthcare system. Although Americans are more likely to believe in God and to go to church than Europeans or East Asians, our healthcare arrangements do not live up to the precepts of our Judeo-Christian heritage. Instead, we have designed a system where people with money or good insurance get great care in great hospitals—while some 30 million others can barely get in the door until they are sick enough to be admitted to the emergency department.

If we had the political will to provide healthcare for everybody, the world's other rich countries could show us the way.

T. R. Reid has become one of the nation's best-known correspondents through his reporting for the Washington Post, NPR, and PBS. His best-selling book The Healing of America *launched him into a national campaign to convince Americans that universal healthcare coverage is a moral imperative. PBS Frontline made two documentaries following Reid as he traveled the world reporting for that book. Reid has written nine books in English and three in Japanese.*

A Call to Action: Harold C. Slavkin

Can you hear the "call"—a call for you to become engaged in your community? If you are reading this essay, it is reasonable to assume that you have had many advantages—affirmative actions by family, friends, and teachers—that enabled you to become all that you have become. In your lifetime, to date, 4.5 million babies were born each year, of which 25 percent were born into extreme poverty, often without hope, dreams, or affirmative actions. Yes, more than 1 million babies each year are born into poverty! These babies will have limited access to early childhood development, preschool programs, K-12 education, and healthcare, and they will have lives replete with chronic diseases and disorders, resulting in reduced life expectancy. Can their fate be changed?

Each of us has many leadership moments in a lifetime—calls to action—to mobilize people to focus on solving problems of significance to the larger society! I am reaching out to you to address the enormous challenge of health disparities and economic inequities throughout America.

Health disparities presents challenges—teenage sexually transmitted diseases, teenage pregnancy, inadequate prenatal care, birth defects (structural and behavioral), child and spousal abuse, childhood obesity, type 1 and 2 diabetes, and an array of chronic diseases and disorders such as cancers; heart, lung, kidney, muscle, bone, and dental diseases and disorders (tooth decay, periodontal disease, and associated tooth loss); and the plight of frail older adults with associated neurovascular diseases. Of course, there are many examples of learning disabilities, behavioral aberrations, and, eventually, limited life expectancy. Today, our nation struggles to address prenatal care issues for all pregnancies, childhood and adult obesity, "the silent epidemic" of tooth decay in poor children of color, autism, cardiovascular diseases, and dementias. Upstream of these health disparities, representing 80 percent of the disease burden as presented by 25 percent of the U.S. population (today approaching 312 million people), is poverty as a result of economic inequalities. In America, research clearly provides evidence that social and educational mobility is easier for some of us than others. It is a cluster of socioeconomic determinants that results in poverty, health disparities, and economic inequalities. Further, we must provide advocacy for the millions of people who are our nation's poor and working poor!

The number one chronic disease of children is tooth decay, and this disease is preventable! Imagine—an American dies every hour from oral cancer, and this chronic disease is also preventable! In fact, most of the major chronic diseases and disorders are preventable through individual choices—choices of diet, exercise, and the avoidance of tobacco products, alcohol, and recreational drug use.

The consequences of economic inequality are profound. Of all industrial nations of the world, U.S. women have the shortest life expectancy, with poor and working poor women of color having the poorest life expectancy statistics.

Imagine the possibilities—economic gains increase our nation's middle class, and that improvement in the human condition results in education, wealth, wellness, and major advances in the quality of life for more people. Can we envision such a nation as a result of our individual enlightened self-interest? Can we envision prenatal care, early childhood development, a superior K-12 education, and multiple postsecondary education options for education and/or training for all people? A higher minimum wage?

Can we achieve a more reasonable distribution of wealth rather than perpetuate the 1 percent wealthy versus the remaining 99 percent? Should the 20 percent of the U.S. population with a college education continue to possess 50 percent of our nation's wealth? Can we close or reduce the gap in wealth between the penthouse and the poorhouse? Should a CEO of a major national industry be compensated 422 times the median compensation for a worker in that industry? Can these and related advances in our civilization also result in a profound decline in violence and killings? Despite remarkable advances in science and technology, we continue to defer social investments that improve the human condition, leave millions of people behind, and devastate the lives and dreams of our children and of our civilization. Income inequality has surged in the United States since the 1970s, and our situation has become much more unequal than Europe. Ironically, despite our nation's alleged science and technology prowess, we spend more money on healthcare, K-12 education, and federal and state welfare programs than any other industrial nation in the world, yet our results rank us among the mediocre nations of the world. In terms of wellness, we rank nineteenth to twenty-first in morbidity and mortality, education attainment in K-12 education, childbirth deaths, tooth loss, and life expectancy. These data sets are particularly valid descriptors for children, adults, and older adults of color—the historically underserved people of America. Can we craft "smart" policies that result in success that really improves quality of life for all people in the United States?

Following World War II, a number of public policies resulted in a rapid expansion of the middle class in the United

States—the GI Bill and higher education opportunities for many millions of returning veterans; land-grant universities; digital and biological research investments through the NIH (National Institutes of Health), NSF (National Science Foundation), and DOD (Department of Defense); civil rights legislation; DHEW (Department of Health, Education and Welfare) programs to address K-12 education; health education and practices; and numerous welfare programs. This so-called Golden Era lasted from 1950 to 1980, triggering an increase in middle-class America and a "pause" in the concentration of wealth in the hands of 1 percent of the nation. Since the 1980s, the middle class has become endangered, the size of the homeless population has grown, and the nation's wealth is increasingly held by 1 percent of our U.S. population.

How will you respond to this call? Our society as a whole is rapidly moving toward knowledge-based economies, with wealth increasingly reflecting level of education and know-how, science and math skills, social skills, appreciation of cultural diversity, and networking. What piece of "wellness" and "economic inequities" will you pursue? We need your energy, intellect, and willingness to stay focused for the long haul. I argue that it is in your enlightened self-interest to contribute to the health, education, and welfare success of those around you in your communities (and beyond). Can we profoundly reduce violence, racism, and poverty while increasing wellness and literacy for all Americans?

Dr. Harold C. Slavkin is currently Professor and Dean Emeritus at the School of Dentistry, University of Southern California, and Board Member for Patterson Companies and The LA Trust for Children's Health. He holds Honorary Degrees from several universities: Peking, Connecticut, Detroit, Maryland, Georgetown, New Jersey, AT Still, and Montreal. He has published many hundreds of scientific papers, 91 invited chapters, and 11 books, including Birth of a Discipline *and his first novel,* Atlanta. *For almost five decades, he has been an advocate for underserved populations to gain access to comprehensive quality healthcare that includes mental, vision, and oral healthcare.*

Free Market Healthcare Reform: Michael Tanner

The Patient Protection and Affordable Care Act is now law, but the debate is far from over. For years to come, we can expect to see continued calls for changes to the landmark law as well at its outright repeal. But those who believe that the ACA, with is centralized "command and control" approach to healthcare reform, is mistaken, have an obligation to suggest alternatives.

The U.S. healthcare system, after all, has much to recommend it. We produce most of the research, innovation, and technology that improves healthcare throughout the world. Americans have more choice of physicians and treatments than patients in other countries. And if you are sick, your chances of survival are far better in this country than elsewhere. But healthcare costs too much. The United States spends more on healthcare than any other industrialized country, nearly a third more than the next highest. At the same time, even after implementation of the ACA, too many Americans lack health insurance or access to needed care.

How, then, can we fix what is wrong with our healthcare system while preserving what is good about it?

First, we need to move away from a system dominated by employer-provided health insurance and instead make health insurance personal and portable, controlled by the individual rather than the government or an employer. There is, after all, no logical reason for individuals to receive health insurance through their jobs. We do not, in fact, receive most other types of insurance—auto, homeowners, life—in that way.

Employer-based health insurance is actually an anomaly that grew out of unique historical circumstances during World War II. Despite the widespread entry of women into the labor force during the war, the shift of men from private employment to the military created a labor shortage. At the same time, wage controls prevented employers from competing for available workers by raising wages. In an effort to circumvent the wage controls and compete for available workers, employers began to offer nonwage benefits, including health insurance. In 1953, the Internal Revenue Service (IRS) ruled that employer-provided health insurance was *not* part of wage compensation for tax purposes.

This means that if a worker is paid $40,000, but their employer also provides an insurance policy worth $10,000, the worker pays taxes on just the $40,000 in wages. If, however, instead of providing insurance, the employer gave the worker a $10,000 raise—allowing the worker to purchase her own insurance—she would have to pay taxes on $50,000. This puts workers who buy their own insurance at a significant disadvantage compared to those who receive insurance through work.

Employment-based insurance seriously distorts our healthcare system in several ways. Most significantly, it hides much of the true cost of healthcare to consumers, thereby encouraging overconsumption.

Imagine someone shopping for groceries under a situation where someone else has agreed to pay 86 percent of whatever the bill turns out to be. That shopper would almost certainly buy more and more expensive food than he would if he were paying the bill himself. There would be a lot more steak and a lot less hamburger. The same holds true for healthcare.

The RAND Health Insurance Experiment, the largest study ever done of consumer health purchasing behavior, provides ample evidence that consumers purchase more healthcare if someone else is paying for it. In particular, families with no co-payment used 53 percent more hospital services (measured in dollars) and had 63 percent more visits for doctors, drugs, and other services than did families with a 95 percent copayment. Overall, the total use of medical resources was 58 percent greater for the group with no copayment, despite virtually identical health outcomes. Even smaller copayment rates produced savings. The study found that an individual with no copayment spent 18 percent more on healthcare than an individual with a 25 percent copayment. Yet, with few exceptions, there was little or no difference in outcomes.

More recently, a study by Amy Finkelstein of MIT suggested that the prevalence of third-party payment in the United States has nearly doubled the cost of healthcare in this country. Finkelstein looked at the U.S. Medicare program for older adults, essentially the largest insurance program for older adults and a program with very low out of pocket costs for participants. She found that the program led to a 23 percent increase in total hospital expenditures (for all ages) between 1965 and 1970. Extrapolating from these estimates, Finkelstein concluded that the overall spread of third-party health insurance between 1950 and 1990 may be responsible for more than 40 percent of the increase in per capita health spending over that period.

Employer-based health insurance also limits consumer choice because employers get the final say in what type of insurance a worker will receive. The entire controversy over whether corporations should be required to include contraceptive coverage in their insurance plans is the result of a system in which insurance is based on your place of employment. A woman who wants an insurance plan that covers contraceptives should be able to take the money that the company is currently paying for insurance and buy the policy that she wants, rather than a plan provided by the employer. The worker gets the coverage she wants, and the company does not have to directly pay for contraceptive coverage that it is morally opposed to. Everyone wins.

Moreover, our current employment-based health insurance system means that people who do not receive insurance through work are put at a significant and costly disadvantage. And, of course, it means that if you lose your job, you are likely to end up uninsured.

Changing from employer to individual insurance requires changing the tax treatment of health insurance. Employer-

provided insurance should be treated the same as other compensation for tax purposes, that is, as taxable income.
To offset the increased tax, workers should receive a standard
deduction, a tax credit, or better still, large Health Savings
Accounts (HSAs) for the purchase of health insurance, regardless of whether they receive it through their job or purchase it
on their own.

As a result of this shift in tax policy, employers would likely
gradually begin to substitute higher wages for insurance,
allowing each worker to shop for the insurance policy that most
closely matches his or her needs. That insurance would be more
likely to be true insurance, protecting the worker against catastrophic risk while requiring out of pocket payment for routine,
low-dollar costs, and it would belong to the worker, not the
employer, meaning that workers would be able to take it from
job to job and would not lose it if they became unemployed.

Putting purchasing power in the hands of consumers is only
half of market-based reform. The other part of effective healthcare reform involves increasing competition among both
insurers and health providers. Current regulations establish
monopolies and cartels in both industries. Today, for example,
people cannot purchase health insurance across state lines. And
because different states have very different regulations and
mandates, costs can vary widely depending on where you live.

New Jersey, for example, requires insurers to cover a wide
range of procedures and types of care, including in vitro fertili-
zation, contraceptives, chiropodists, and coverage of children
until they reach age 25. Those mandated benefits are not
cheap. According to a 2006 analysis by the National Center
for Policy Analysis, the cost of a standard health insurance policy for a healthy 25-year-old man averaged $5,580 in the state.
A standard policy in Kentucky, which has far fewer mandates,
would cost the same man only $960 per year.

Unfortunately, consumers are more or less held prisoner by
their state's regulatory regime. It is illegal for that hypothetical
New Jersey resident to buy the cheaper health insurance in

Kentucky. On the other hand, if consumers were free to purchase insurance in other states, they could in effect "purchase" the regulations of that other state. A consumer in New Jersey could avoid the state's regulatory costs and choose, say, Kentucky, if that state's regulations aligned more closely with his or her preferences.

With millions of American consumers balancing costs and risks, states would be forced to evaluate whether their regulations offered true value or simply reflected the influence of special interests.

We also need to rethink medical licensing laws to encourage greater competition among providers. Nurse practitioners, physician assistants, midwives, and other nonphysician practitioners should have far greater ability to treat patients. We also should be encouraging such innovations in delivery as medical clinics in retail outlets.

All of this is designed to put consumers in charge of the healthcare system. After all, it is individual consumers demanding better quality at a lower price that makes markets in other goods and services work. Consider computers. Not so long ago, computers were the size of a house and were so expensive only universities or big businesses could own them. Today, there is one in your cell phone. That is the power of consumer control.

We can do the same thing with healthcare.

Michael Tanner is a senior fellow with the Cato Institute in Washington, DC, and co-author of Healthy Competition: What's Holding Back Healthcare and How to Free It.

Basic Health Access: Robert C. Bowman

Numerous articles indicate physician shortages. There is general agreement that there are particular shortages of certain physicians by specialty or by type of location. While it is common to think that primary care shortages are a more recent event, primary care deficits have been persistent for decades. Short-term deficits suggest short-term solution focus.

Deficits across an entire generation of workforce point to failures in the designs that shape workforce—training design and payment design.

Articles about primary care solutions regularly appear. Most claim that new payment designs, new software, new types of clinicians, or reorgananizations of care will solve primary care deficits. Innovations, reforms, and reorganizations do not have the specific focus on clinicians and teams needed. This is why primary care delivery deficits will remain for the coming generation of workforce as in the last generation, from 1980 to the present.

Physician training is an example of exactly the wrong design to address primary care deficits. Residency training is the last and most important influence of physician training with regard to physician practice location. The U.S. design for residency training:

- Concentrates residency training in the six states that have the highest concentrations of physicians
- Focuses training locations at sites with the highest concentrations of physicians
- Emphasizes specialties, subspecialties, and subsubspecialties other than primary care

Studies by Chen and colleagues indicate the failure of legislated graduate medical education (GME) reform to shift residency training positions to states most in need of physicians, and to training where workforce is needed, such as rural areas have made the shortage of primary care physicians even worse (Chen 2013).

These three dimensions are exactly the opposite of what is required to recover health access:

1. *Instate for 30 states behind by design.* Resident training is a 20–40 times multiplier of physician instate practice location as compared to less than 5 times greater for instate

birth or for instate medical school. Training design fails for 30 states in need of physicians and favors 6 states with top concentrations. The economic impact of medical education indicates much the same with $250 billion, or half of the economic impact, specific to six states. (Association of American Medical Colleges, 2008)

2. *Practice location outside of concentrations of physicians.* Zip code locations of residents in the AMA Masterfile indicate that 85 percent of residents are found in 3,400 zip codes where only 35 percent of Americans are found. Only 15 percent of training occurs in 40,000 zip codes outside of concentrations of physicians where Americans are older, less healthy, less wealthy, less educated, and face gaps in services and resources. (Medical Marketing Service, 2013)

3. *More primary care graduates that also remain in primary care for a career.* As Jolly noted in *Academic Medicine*, subsubspecialty fellowships created by teaching hospitals and filled by candidates have increased at 11 percent per year for the past decade. Subspecialty positions filled have increased by 4 percent each year. With more specialties created and more subcategories added to each specialty, fewer physicians remain in core specialties, including primary care specialties. Resolution of health access requires production of core specialties—the ones most important for rural areas and all locations with lower concentrations of clinicians.

Nurse practitioner and physician assistant graduates have followed the same pattern. This is another indication that all sources of clinicians are shaped similarly by payment policy.

The movement to greater specialization favors teaching hospitals and the fellows and their employers, but there are consequences, including declines in primary care results, basic specialties, and distribution.

Internal medicine is a primary example of decline by design. Internal medicine training was once the largest source of primary care physicians. For decades of class years, internal medicine training resulted in over 3,000 annual graduates per year found in office general internal medicine. This can be multiplied by 35 class years (one generation of class years) for a result of over 100,000 in the primary care workforce. The office primary care result from each class year has declined below 1,500 internal medicine graduates for class years since 1998. This translates to internal medicine office primary care cut in half to less than 50,000 internal medicine primary care physicians by 2030 or sooner. Internal medicine has sustained losses of 30,000 becoming hospitalists in recent years (Medicine, S.o.H.2014).

Internal medicine is the best indicator of reward for specialization, as IM has also shown the most decline, from over 50 percent office primary care in the 1990s to less than 20 percent (Hauer, 2008; West and Dupras, 2012). Losses of internal medicine primary care physicians were devastating from 2010 to 2040—a time with the largest increase in adult and senior primary care demand.

Family medicine has become the top source of the physician workforce and has consistently been the most important source where primary care is lower to lowest in concentrations of clinicians. This is reflected in a rural workforce in which family physicians comprise 25 percent compared to internal medicine primary care at 12 percent and pediatrics at 6 percent (Medical Marketing Service, 2013).

Unfortunately, the training design interacts with payment policy to prevent the choice of a permanent primary care choice such as family medicine. Medical school admission choices and training influences erect a barrier to permanent primary care. It is difficult to choose FM when health policy is poorly supportive of primary care and care where needed—the locations favored by family physicians.

Pediatrics is also stagnant for primary care results and represents a distant third most important rural workforce, or about 6 percent of the primary care workforce where needed.

Expansions of pediatric training no longer increase primary care results. The same annual 1,400 office primary care pediatricians per class year have remained despite an increase in annual graduates from 2,200 to 2,800 from 1980 to the present (Medical Marketing Service, 2013).

An optimal result for training would be over 80 percent of graduates retained in primary care, with all training in the state in need of clinicians and training location influences specific to areas in need of clinicians in the state. Family medicine medical schools with preparation, admission, all training, and obligation would align instate, permanent primary care, and where needed.

Nurse practitioners and physician assistants could also meet this optimal result, but this would require additional regulation to result in 80 percent family practice position results for a career—the opposite policy direction as compared to the last 50 years. Flexible designs allow graduates of all clinician sources to be free to follow spending design to states with greater health spending, to nonprimary care specialties with better payment support, and to locations with higher concentrations of workforce (Bowman, 2008, 2010).

A design specific to primary care recovery must avoid distractions. Two distractions in the past decade have captured two large chunks of primary care trained clinicians. The new specialty of hospital medicine has resulted in the loss of over 40,000 primary care trained physicians. Resident work hours limitations have left a gap in teaching hospital clinicians that has been filled by tens of thousands of nurse practitioners and physician assistants.

Regardless of the health professional training situation, primary care recovery can only occur with improved support for primary care. This must involve increases in revenue, decreases in cost of delivery, or both. At the current time the primary care revenue is stagnant or declining and the cost of delivery is increasing rapidly. The same mechanisms preventing rural workforce are also preventing primary care workforce (Bowman, 2014).

To understand primary care deficits, it is important to understand the financial challenges within primary care practices. This is most important for the small primary care practices that are 45 percent of primary care in the United States (Alaskan Center for Rural Health, 2006). More personnel are required to address regulations, screen patients, address billing problems (denial, delay), improve quality, manage costly patients, and beg insurance payers for care for their patients (prescription approvals, access to specialists, hospital admission, etc.). The designs for the payment process require primary care offices to make investments that save dollars for someone else. Smaller providers cannot get cost breaks for supplies or insurance and may end up paying more because of discounts given to the largest health operations who demand and get discounts. Incentive costs for recruitment and retention as well as locums costs are rising. Each cost increase not specific to the clinicians and team members that deliver care is a cost that dilute primary care delivery. The situation is even more difficult for care where needed where small practices and complex patients dominate care.

Health access recovery requires specific changes in training and in payment that are specific to states in need, primary care, and locations in need of clinicians.

References

Alaskan Center for Rural Health. (2006). *Anchorage, Alaska Center for Rural Health, University of Alaska, Anchorage, 2005–2006.*

Association of American Medical Colleges. (2008). *The Economic Impact of AAMC-Member Medical Schools and Teaching Hospitals.* Washington, DC: Association of American Medical Colleges.

Bowman, R. C. (2010). *The Standard Primary Care Year Web Site.* http://www.ruralmedicaleducation.org/basichealthaccess/The_Standard_Primary_Care_Year.htm.

Bowman, R. C. (2008). Measuring Primary Care: The Standard Primary Care Year. *Rural Remote Health* 8(3).

Bowman, R. C., and M. P. Halasy. (2014). Preventing Rural Workforce by Design. *Rural Remote Health* 14(2): 2852.

Chen, C. et al. (2013). Toward Graduate Medical Education (GME) Accountability: Measuring the Outcomes of GME Institutions. *Academic Medicine* 88(9): 1267–1280.

Hauer, K. E. et al. (2008). Factors Associated with Medical Students' Career Choices Regarding Internal Medicine. *JAMA* 300(10): 1154–1164.

Medical Marketing Service. (2013). *AMA Physician Masterfile*. http://www.mmslists.com.

State of Hospital Medicine. (2014). Philadelphia: SHM: Society of Hospital Medicine.

West, C. P., and D. M. Dupras. (2012). General Medicine vs Subspecialty Career Plans among Internal Medicine Residents. *JAMA* 308(21): 2241–2247.

Robert C. Bowman, MD, School of Osteopathic Medicine in Arizona, A. T. Still University of the Health Sciences

Critiquing Consumer-Driven Healthcare: Greg Shaw

As employers, governments, and families struggle to confront the reality that Americans will spend over 17 percent of our GDP on health expenses in 2014, one of the more lively conversations among experts addresses strategies to incentivize patients to behave more like competitive shoppers in healthcare markets. Toward this goal, the consumer-driven healthcare movement advocates policies that more fully expose individuals to the costs of the health services they obtain with the expectation that this greater transparency will lead to more price sensitivity, more selective use of health goods and services, and a sharper focus on purchasing highly effective treatments.

Consisting mainly of cost-sharing provisions, these policy pre-scriptions can claim some evidentiary support. However, they also engender much debate. This essay considers some of the limitations to the consumer-driven healthcare (CDHC) move-ment, both in terms of the fiscal effectiveness of cost-sharing and the normative complaints about such practices.

The most comprehensive study of consumer-driven health-care is the widely cited RAND Corporation project of the late 1970s and early 1980s. Participants were randomly assigned to various copayment categories, ranging from zero to 95 per-cent. Among its findings were that participants displayed price sensitivity, with those in the free healthcare condition consum-ing 4.25 percent more than those persons in the 25 percent copay group and 45 percent more than those in the 95 percent copay group.

While many have found these results compelling, others have critiqued the CDHC movement over its efficacy and normative implications. Broadly, cost-sharing provisions—such as elevated copayments and health savings accounts (HSAs)—most lend themselves to individuals and families with ample disposable income. As the RAND study found, individ-uals who are both sick and poor fared significantly worse under that experiment than did others. Paying the increased copay-ments and deductibles or contributing to an HSA is clearly more viable for those with discretionary income. For their part, employers have increasingly embraced HSAs as a way to limit their own financial liability for their employees' health expenses. This effort to shift greater responsibility to individ-uals and away from firms has achieved some success, as over 15 million Americans currently own an HSA.

Cost-sharing turns out to be something of a blunt instru-ment when implemented broadly. These provisions adversely affect individuals whom they require to shoulder directly a greater portion of their health expenses. Evidence suggests that low-income persons respond to these requirements by deferring preventative care. Further, because approximately 10 percent of the nation's population is responsible for approximately 70 percent of the nation's health expenditures (and the healthiest 50 percent of the population is responsible for only about 3 percent of health costs), applying cost-sharing imposes costs on a large portion of the population that is not particularly responsible for rising system-wide costs (Jost 2007).

Cost-sharing also fails to lead consumers to select the most effective treatments. According to the RAND Corporation study, participants who faced copayments did not systematically tend to elect more effective over less effective treatments. Similarly, while participants did reduce the number of office visits in line with their rising copayment level, once in the doctor's office, these individuals did not reduce the number of services they consumed in relation to their copayment level. This strongly suggests that at least as much of the responsibility for cost cutting lies with medical professionals as with patients. The old saying that the most expensive piece of equipment in a hospital is the doctor's pen—and with it, his or her ability to order services to be rendered—still seems to prevail.

The consumer-driven perspective extends the moral hazard argument to claim that many people engage in risky behaviors because they have too much health insurance. If individuals had to pay out of pocket instead, so this argument goes, they would lead healthier lives. As it turns out, the evidence for risky behavior supposedly induced by ample health insurance is weak (Jost 2007). Whether or not it is moral to ask taxpayers to help pay for public programs, such as Medicare and Medicaid, to cover the health costs for people who have neglected their health is, of course, bound up with the broader argument about how these two programs also fund services for individuals who have paid taxes and who are of average health. In the end, arguing that a significant portion of the population creates a problem by having too much insurance may prove difficult for politicians, given the tens of millions of Americans who still lack insurance coverage.

One particularly attractive target for CDHC advocates is the very expensive Medicare program, a piece of the safety net that benefits over 50 million people but carries costs that will top $600 billion in 2015. Given Medicare's expenditures, turning it into a voucher program is viewed by some as an opportunity to encourage older adults to shop for the cheapest insurance available, to not buy too much of it, and to lead healthier lives. Of course, this perspective arguably underappreciates the need for basic medical services. Purchasing healthcare is unlike purchasing luxury goods. A common image in the consumer-driven literature is to compare first-dollar health insurance coverage to first-dollar coverage for housing or restaurant meals. The criticism from the CDHC perspective is that having such insurance encourages overutilization. Of course, this comparison ignores the reality that health services are usually inconvenient, unpleasant, uncomfortable, and sometimes just plain painful. A small minority of individuals may seek services in excess, but most people have better things to do.

Finally, comparing patients to haggling shoppers strains credibility in many quarters. In the words of one physician interviewed in McAllen, Texas, in 2009 who quipped about such a negotiation: "A cardiologist tells an elderly woman that she needs bypass surgery and had Dr. Dyke see her. They discuss the blockages in her heart, the operation, [and] the risks. And now they're supposed to haggle over the price as if he were selling a rug in a souk? 'I'll do three vessels for thirty thousand, but if you take four I'll throw in an extra night in the I.C.U.'— that sort of thing? Dyke shook his head. 'Who comes up with this stuff?' he asked. 'Any plan that relies on the sheep to negotiate with the wolves is doomed to failure' " (Gawande, 2009).

References

Gawande, Atul. (2009, June 1). "The Cost Conundrum: What a Texas Town Can Teach Us about Healthcare." *New Yorker*. http://www.newyorker.com/magazine/2009/06/01/the-cost-conundrum.

Jost, Timothy. (2007). *Healthcare at Risk.* Durham, NC: Duke University Press.

Greg Shaw, Professor and Chair, Department of Political Science, Illinois Wesleyan University

Why U.S.-Style Health Reform Does Not Work and What to Do about It: Claudia Chaufan

The Story of Teresa

Teresa (I have changed the name of the protagonist of this story to protect her privacy) came to me in tears. The stack of bills—including hospital, doctors, and ambulance services claims—added up to slightly under $20,000, over a year's worth of her income. "Believe me, Dr. Claudia, I felt like I was going to die, like my abdomen would explode. I was so scared . . ." she said. "I barely managed to call my daughter, who saw me in that state and called the ambulance," she continued, adding almost apologetically: "I can assure you she gave the medics my insurance card. But they didn't look at it. They just took me to that clinic."

At the clinic, Teresa was rushed to the emergency department, where, as she relayed to me, medical personnel inserted an intravenous line (IV), performed a physical examination, ordered tests, and determined that her condition—likely due to a ruptured ovarian cyst—was stable. The whole ordeal took about four hours, including the time Teresa was kept under observation until she felt better, after which she left the hospital with a prescription for painkillers and instructions to follow up with her doctor.

So why those bills? Is Teresa uninsured? No, she is not. Is she an undocumented immigrant? No. She has a green card and is on her way to becoming a citizen. Yet, she is out of luck because her coverage is skimpy. She does not qualify for Medicaid (Medical in California), not because California shunned the Medicaid expansion, but because she makes too much money to meet Medicaid's income eligibility criteria. And the plan she can afford, even with subsidies, requires that she shoulder 40 percent her medical bills. And it does not help that Teresa's plan does not include the providers and medical establishments where the ambulance took her.

Five months after the documented "date of service," I am still struggling to convince Teresa's providers that she cannot pay her bills upfront, not even with a "generous" discount (50 percent). Nor can she afford to be debt bound by monthly payments. Her children and grandchildren count on her economic support back in Latin America. So I have helped her fill out about 15 pages of forms, collect financial and other documentation, and file for "charitable care."

Incidentally, I have a medical degree and a PhD in sociology, and more years of education than I want to remember (or confess). I still fail to understand the "explanation of benefits," which I requested to sort out Teresa's coverage. Am I a case of "low health literacy"—described in leading medical journals (Sentell 2012) and official websites (DHHS 2014) as a "major" impediment to successful reform—unusual given my socioeconomic status? Do I need a "navigator"? (Kaiser Foundation, 2013). But I digress. I will spare readers other shocking details of Teresa's case. I suspect she is not alone (most Americans saddled by medical debt to the point of filing for bankruptcy have insurance).

Health Policy Hypes and (False) Hopes

Let me move on instead to examine whether the "solutions" usually proposed to the problems of restricted access, deteriorating quality, and spiraling costs—critical features of U.S. healthcare even after the implementation of major reform (Davis 2007, 2010; Davis 2014; Commonwealth Fund 2006; Thomson 2013)—would have helped Teresa. I will focus on electronic health records, medical homes, price transparency, and wellness programs (there are many others, like health savings accounts, pay-for-performance, etc., but I will set those aside).

Would electronic health records have helped Teresa? Not really. In fact, Teresa's health information is carefully kept in an electronic health record in a medical home—her family doctor at an "in-network" clinic that is her usual source of care. But it is not there that the ambulance chose to take Teresa. In fact, neither Teresa nor her daughter speaks very good English, and the medics did not speak Spanish, and at any rate, they had tasks more urgent than figuring out whether the nearest medical establishment was in Teresa's "network."

What about price transparency? In all honesty, Teresa's bills were anything but "transparent." But what if they had been? Well, I think Teresa was in no position to comparison shop for prices, however transparent (nor were the medics on her behalf). Even at sharply discounted rates, those prices would be just too high for her. Nor, I imagine, was she in a position to challenge the doctors' judgment about the "cost-effectiveness" of the services received (nor, in my opinion, should she be required to). I will not bother the reader with the potential usefulness of wellness programs for this occasion. One does not need to be an expert to understand that they are irrelevant when dealing with a ruptured ovarian cyst.

So what, if anything, would have helped Teresa? Well, in my view, it would have helped her if she had been a Canadian immigrant, living under a single-payer system.

What Is Single Payer?

Single-payer national health insurance is a system in which a single public or quasi-public agency (or strictly regulated subsidiaries) organizes healthcare financing, that is, collects the money from users, purchases services in bulk, and negotiates rates and payment schemes with, and pays, providers. The delivery of care may remain or not in private hands. Nations that have adopted single-payer systems cut across cultures, political ideologies, and levels of development. They include countries as different as the United Kingdom, Iceland, Taiwan, Spain, and Cuba. In fact, all wealthy nations with the exception of the United States, and many poor nations, have organized their healthcare systems as variants of single payer (Chaufan 2011).

The Expanded and Improved Medicare for All Act, HR 676, based on a physicians' proposal crafted by members of Physicians for a National Health Program and published in *JAMA*, would establish an American single-payer health insurance system (Woolhandler and Himmelstein 2002).

Under this system, all residents, documented or not, would be covered for all medically necessary services, including doctor, hospital, preventive, long-term care, mental health, reproductive healthcare, dental, vision, prescription drugs, and medical supplies. Dramatic overall savings would ensue from the system's power to purchase goods and services in bulk and thus negotiate prices with providers' associations, pharmaceutical companies, and medical device suppliers. Paper pushing that does not contribute to more or better care—preapprovals, approvals, marketing, determination of patient eligibility for services on the part of insurers and providers, denials, appeals—would be eliminated, and so would overpayments to private (Advantage) Medicare plans. Collectively, savings would amount to around $600 billion annually, more than enough to provide first dollar coverage for every U.S. resident (Friedman 2013; Hellander, Himmelstein, and Woolhandler 2013).

Even though taxes might slightly increase, most Americans would save money, time, and distress, as they would no longer be compelled to comparison shop for increasingly pricier and inscrutable plans, juggle with unpredictable (and unaffordable) out of pocket costs (premiums and out of pocket costs would disappear), or struggle to figure out which providers are "in network," as most providers in the country would find it convenient to join the system (See Table 3.1).

Table 3.1.   Comparing Gains under ACA and Single Payer

	ACA	Single Payer
Universal Coverage	NO. More than 30 million remain uninsured (mostly citizens and documented residents) by 2024 and tens of millions underinsured	YES. Everybody is covered automatically at birth
Full Range of Benefits	NO. HHS provides "guidance" on "essential health benefits"; what counts as benefits decided on the basis of existing plans, i.e., by insurers themselves	YES. Covered for all medically necessary care
Choice of Doctors and Hospitals	NO. Insurance companies continue to restrict access through increasingly narrower networks of "preferred" (by them!) providers	YES. Patients can choose among any participating provider; most providers in the country would find it convenient to participate
Out of Pocket	YES. Varying degrees of copays and deductibles; trade-offs between lower premiums (even if ever increasing) and higher out of pocket expenses via "consumer-directed" plans	NO. Copays and deductibles eliminated
Savings	NO. Increases health spending by about $1.1 trillion	YES. Redirects $600 billion in administrative waste and inflated drug prices toward care; no net increase in health spending
Cost-Control/ Sustainability	NO. Preserves a fragmented system incapable of controlling costs; gains in coverage erased by rising out of pocket expenses, bureaucratic waste, and profiteering by private insurers and big pharma	YES. Large-scale cost controls through econo-mies of scale to ensure that benefits are sustain-able over the long term
Progressive Financing	NO. Costs are disproportionately paid by middle- and lower-income Americans and those families fac-ing acute or chronic illness	YES. Premiums and out of pocket costs are replaced with progressive income and wealth taxes; 95 percent of Americans pay less

Sources:

1. Physicians for a National Health Program (PNHP). (2014, August 1). *A Superior System: Single Payer Legislation vs. Affordable Care Act.* http://www.pnhp.org/sites/default/files/docs/2010/Single-Payer-Reconciliation-Comparison-Table.pdf.

2. Congressional Budget Office (CBO). (2014). *Insurance Coverage Provisions of the Affordable Care Act: CBO's April 2014 Baseline.* http://www.cbo.gov/sites/default/files/cbofiles/attachments/43900-2014-04-ACAtables2.pdf.

But, Isn't Single Payer "Un-American"?

As a matter of fact, the United States has close to 50 years of experience with single-payer-like programs. One such case is Medicare, the publicly financed plan for older adults and persons with disabilities. Compared to the rocky rollout of the Affordable Care Act (ACA), the beginnings of Medicare were rather uneventful. Less than a year into becoming the law of the land in 1965, Medicare was paying the medical bills of over 19 million older adults (99 percent of those eligible for coverage) (SSA 2013)—with no websites, navigators, or the threat of financial penalties.

Because most seniors were already known to the Social Security Administration, Social Security numbers were used to enroll them for hospital services (Part A), and index cards were used for doctors' services (Part B). As a national social insurance program administered by the U.S. federal government, Medicare granted older adults full rights to the same comprehensive package of services and free choice of any participating provider. As a public program, it dispensed with the pursuit of profit, which is the lifeblood of commercial insurance, so the costs of marketing or of helping users navigate "coverage options"—substantial with the ACA (CaliforniaHealthine April 2013, May 2013)—were zero.

Providers gained independence in medical decision-making and the guarantee that their bills would get paid. There was, and there remains, much room for improvement—in access, coverage, quality, and cost control. But the relevant feature of Medicare was, and remains, its financial structure; the program is organized as a social insurance system. Social insurance spreads financial risk associated with illness across society to protect everyone. Enrollees pay according to their ability and are entitled to the same comprehensive package of services according to their medical needs. In contrast, the individual mandate, which requires millions of Americans to purchase a commercial product—heavily subsidized by taxpayers[1]—and is the cornerstone of the ACA, has no precedent in U.S. history.

The Way Forward

As President Obama correctly pointed out, you can have universal coverage—and I would add no ugly surprises with unpayable medical bills for you or your loved ones—and you can have lower costs, but you need single-payer to have both. In fact, a mere three years before becoming a senator, Obama was on record supporting single payer. Sadly, as he advanced in his political career, he had a change of heart (*Barack Obama Promotes* 2013)—which is a topic for another article.

As Dr. Margaret Flowers, a pediatrician, and Kevin Zeese, an attorney and corporate watchdog, persuasively argue, there is reason to believe that what is now the law of the land will do little to put a check on the big drivers of the rising cost of U.S. healthcare—insurance conglomerates, big pharma, for-profit hospitals—which will necessarily undermine any attempt to provide equitable access to quality healthcare (Zeese and Flowers 2013). So I will close with their words:

> There was an easier, more politically popular route [than the ACA]. All that President Obama had to do was to push for what he once [said he] believed in, Medicare for All. By dropping two words, "over 65," the country could

---

[1]Taxpayers subsidize commercial health insurers in more than one way. These include (1) direct assistance for users to purchase "insurance products," (2) foregone revenues (i.e., certain payments to insurers are considered nontaxable income), and (3) enrolling sicker or poorer (usually both) segments of the population that insurers find unprofitable. In this latter case, often insurers will "accept" to take on this less profitable population in exchange for generous incentives. This is the case of private Medicare (Advantage) plans, which between 1985 and 2012 received around $300 billion, some 25 percent, over and above the cost of traditional (nonprivatized) Medicare.

have gradually improved Medicare [and moved the country] toward the best healthcare in the world, rather than being mired at the bottom.

I could not agree more. I also agree with them that the task is to organize a mass movement that refuses to treat healthcare as a commodity like a cellphone and recognizes that ending the corporate domination of healthcare is part of breaking the domination of the corporate class over our government and our lives. If we do, we can recover our health, our democracy, and our dignity.

References

Barack Obama Promotes Single-Payer Universal Healthcare (2013, October 20). https://www.youtube.com/watch?v=BKkTRMEyAhs.

CaliforniaHealthline. (2013, May 10). *HHS Offers $150M to Boost Enrollment in State Health Exchanges.* http://www.californiahealthline.org/articles/2013/5/10/hhs-announces-program-to-enroll-uninsured-in-state-health-exchanges.

CaliforniaHealthline. (2013, April 13). *Calif. Health Exchange to Spend $290M on Public Outreach Efforts.* http://www.californiahealthline.org/articles/2013/4/26/calif-health-exchange-to-spend-290m-on-public-outreach-efforts.

Chaufan, C. (2011). Influences of Policy on Healthcare of Families. In M. J. Craft-Rosenberg (Ed.), *Encyclopedia of Family Health*, pp. 650–658. Newbury Park, CA: SAGE.

Commonwealth Fund Commission on a High Performance Health System. (2006, September). *Why Not the Best? Results from a National Scorecard on U.S. Health System Performance.* http://www.commonwealthfund.org/Publications/Fund-Reports/2006/Sep/Why-Not-the-Best—Results-from-a-National-Scorecard-on-U-S—Health-System-Performance.aspx#citation.

Davis, K. et al. (2014). *Mirror, Mirror on the Wall, 2014 Update: How the U.S. Healthcare System Compares Internationally.* Commonwealth Fund. http://www.common wealthfund.org/~/media/files/publications/fund-report/2014/jun/1755_davis_mirror_mirror_2014.pdf.

Davis, K. et al. (2007, May). *Mirror, Mirror on the Wall: An International Update on the Comparative Performance of American Healthcare.* Commonwealth Fund. http://www. commonwealthfund.org/Publications/Fund-Reports/2007/May/Mirror—Mirror-on-the-Wall—An-International-Update-on-the-Comparative-Performance-of-American-Healt.aspx#citation.

Davis, K., C. Schoen, and K. Stremikis. (2010). *Mirror, Mirror on the Wall: How the Performance of the U.S. Healthcare System Compares Internationally, 2010 Update.* Common wealth Fund. http://www.commonwealthfund.org/Publications/Fund-Reports/2010/Jun/Mirror-Mirror-Update.aspx?page=all.

Friedman, G. (2013). *Funding HR 676: The Expanded and Improved Medicare for All Act: How We Can Afford a National Single-Payer Health Plan.* http://www.pnhp.org/sites/default/files/Funding percent20HR percent20676_Friedman_final_7.31.13.pdf.

Hellander, I., D. Himmelstein, and S. Woolhandler. (2013). Medicare Overpayments to Private Plans, 1985–2012: Shifting Seniors to Private Plans Has Already Cost Medicare US$282.6 Billion. *International Journal of Health Service* 43 (2): 305–319.

Kaiser Family Foundation. (2013). *Navigator and In-Person Assistance Programs: A Snapshot of State Programs.* http://kaiserfamilyfoundation.files.wordpress.com/2013/04/8437.pdf.

Physicians for a National Health Program. (2008). *What Is Single Payer?* http://www.pnhp.org/facts/what-is-single-payer.

Sentell, T. (2012). Implications for Reform: Survey of California Adults Suggests Low Health Literacy Predicts Likelihood of Being Uninsured. *Health Affairs* 31(5): 1039–1048.

Social Security Administration (SSA). (2013). *Social Security History.* http://www.ssa.gov/history/ssa/lbjmedicare3.html.

Thomson, S. et al. (2013). *International Profiles of Healthcare Systems.* Commonwealth Fund. http://www.common wealthfund.org/Publications/Fund-Reports/2013/Nov/ International-Profiles-of-Health-Care-Systems.aspx.

U.S. Department of Health and Human Services (DHHS). (2014). *Quick Guide to Health Literacy.* http://www.health .gov/communication/literacy/quickguide/Quickguide.pdf.

Woolhandler, S., and D. U. Himmelstein. (2002). Paying for National Health Insurance—And Not Getting It. *Health Affairs* 21(4): 88–98.

Zeese, K., and M. Flowers. (2013). Obamacare: The Biggest Insurance Scam in History. Truthout. http://www.truth -out.org/opinion/item/19692-obamacare-the-biggest -insurance-scam-in-history.

Claudia Chaufan, MD, PhD, Associate Professor, Institute for Health & Aging

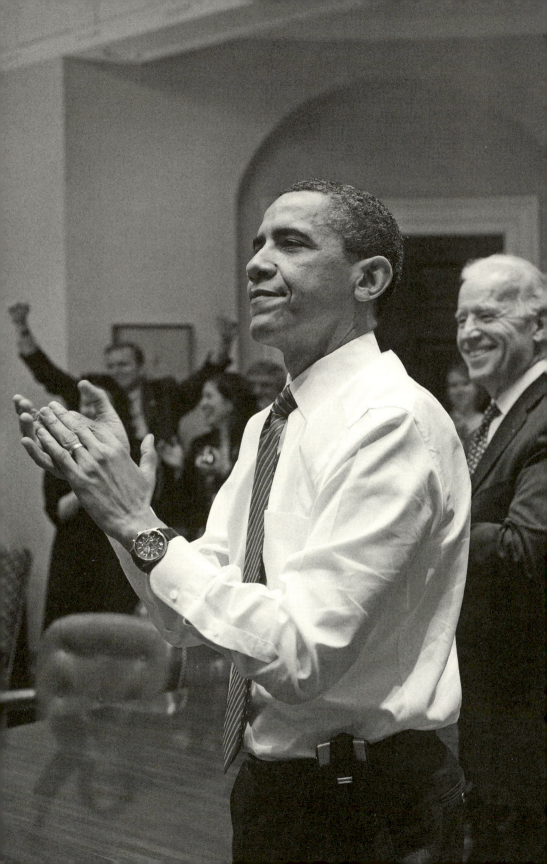

This chapter contains brief sketches of individuals and organizations who are important in understanding healthcare reform in the United States. Only some especially significant organizations and individuals, or those typical of other organizations and individuals, are included.

People

This section provides brief biographical sketches of a number of important men and women in the field of healthcare reform, including those who worked for or against passage of important legislation.

John Boehner (November 17, 1949–)

John Boehner serves as speaker of the U.S. House of Representatives. He was first elected to represent the Eighth Congressional District of Ohio in 1990 and was reelected for a twelfth term in November 2012. He has become a national leader in the drive for a smaller, less costly, and more accountable federal government.

President Barack Obama, Vice President Joe Biden, and senior staff, react in the Roosevelt Room of the White House, as the House passes the healthcare reform bill on March 21, 2010. (The White House)

Boehner has lived in southwest Ohio his entire life and put himself through Xavier University. Before his interest in politics, he ran a small business in the plastics and packaging industry. His political career began with activities in his neighborhood homeowners association, followed by a seat on his township board of trustees and the Ohio General Assembly in 1984. With a focus on reform, he adopted a "no earmarks" policy and then became part of the "Gang of Seven," a group of Republican lawmakers that took on the House establishment, and paid attention to solving the House banking scandal. In 1994, he was one of the authors of the Contract with America. Once Republicans won their first congressional majority in several decades, he was elected to serve as House GOP conference chairman in the 104th and 105th Congresses and became a powerful person in the fight to force Washington to stick to spending limits imposed by the Balanced Budget Act. In 2006, John was elected by his colleagues to serve as House majority leader. During that time, the House passed the first budget that held the line on spending in several years and adopted reforms making the earmark process open and accountable.

In his role as House majority leader, he united Republicans against a number of Obama's proposals such as the Affordable Care Act and the Democrats' "cap and trade" national energy tax. Under his leadership, Republicans launched several efforts to develop solutions to the challenges facing families and small businesses such as the GOP State Solutions project, an initiative aimed at bringing reform-minded Republicans at the state and federal levels together to promote common-sense solutions from outside the Beltway. He was part of the creation of the innovative America Speaking Out project, which gave Americans a platform to discuss and share their priorities with national leaders—a platform that led to the Pledge to America, the Republicans' new governing agenda for the country. First as the minority leader and now as the speaker of the House, he has led the Republican Party's opposition to healthcare reform proposed by Obama in the House of Representatives. The legislation was passed over his objections.

Hillary Rodham Clinton (October 26, 1947–)

Hillary Rodham Clinton is the wife of Bill Clinton, the forty-second president of the United States. A native of Chicago with a law degree from Yale, she was the first First Lady to have her own career before the election of her husband as president. Earlier, when her husband was governor of Arkansas, she also broke ground there by remaining active as a lawyer in addition to being the governor's wife. She also became involved in one of his major policy efforts as governor, the improvement of the public education system in the state of Arkansas.

Clinton served as a key policy advisor to her husband when he was president, and this led to some controversy and concerns about her unofficial role. Some of her work was official, and she led the failed effort in 1993–1994 to pass comprehensive reform of the U.S. healthcare system during Bill Clinton's presidency. This failure was largely the result of lack of experience in national politics of both Clintons. Much of the development of the plan was done without significant input from key congressional leaders. While there was a process of input that included industry leaders, health policy analysts, and government officials, this group was not able to reach consensus about a proposal quickly enough to ensure the emergence of a strong enough coalition to lead to its passage. For the rest of her husband's presidency, she adopted a somewhat lower profile, although her interests in politics remained strong.

Clinton was elected to the U.S. Senate from New York in 2000 and reelected in 2006. After her unsuccessful run for the Democratic presidential nomination in 2008, she accepted a position in President Obama's cabinet as secretary of state and served in that position during the first Obama administration. She made many trips overseas, as is typical for a secretary of state, but seemed to have even more trips and activities abroad than had some previous secretaries of state. While on many of these trips, she spoke out about some of her most passionate interests, including her special concern for women and children and health.

After resigning as secretary of state, she became active in the Clinton Foundation, whose focus includes such concerns as improving global health, increasing opportunity for women and girls, reducing childhood obesity and preventable diseases, creating economic opportunity and growth, and bringing attention to issues of climate change.

William (Bill) Jefferson Clinton (August 19, 1946–)

Bill Clinton was the forty-second president of the United States, serving from 1993 to 2001. He was the third youngest person to be elected president and was known as a dynamic politician who was able to connect with people on a personal level. He showed an early interest in politics and was elected to Boys State while in high school, where he was able to briefly meet one of his political idols, President John Kennedy. He won a prestigious Rhodes Scholarship and through that attended Oxford University in England for two years. He was the first Democrat since Franklin Roosevelt to be elected to a second term. Before running as president, he was the attorney general and then governor of Arkansas. One of his efforts there was to improve the education system in the state.

A major promise in his first campaign for president in 1992 was to enact major reform in the U.S. healthcare system that would ensure access to all while controlling costs. He appointed his wife, Hillary, to lead the effort to develop and enact a national healthcare proposal but was unsuccessful. He was noted for economic success and for some successful efforts in world peace such as in Serbia. After the 1994 healthcare reform failure, and the subsequent loss of control of the House of Representatives to the Republican Party, Clinton declared the era of big government over and changed his focused to making incremental change in government programs, including those related to health. One of the subsequent health reform programs passed included CHIP (Child Health Insurance Program). This program provides health insurance to children of the working poor and near poor, and represented the largest expansion of direct government programs to provide health insurance coverage to Americans since the passage of Medicare and Medicaid in 1965. He also helped pass the Family and Medical Leave Act, which gives many Americans the right to take leave for family needs such as pregnancy or the care of older relatives.

His terms as president were marked with government shutdowns over budget issues and challenges to his presidency based on personal actions, such as his relationship with White House intern Monica Lewinsky. Because of this, he became the second sitting president to be impeached by the House of Representatives, but he was not convicted by the Senate and thus remained in office. Despite these distractions and problems, he left office with reasonable levels of popularity and quickly became involved in some new challenges through the creation of the Clinton Foundation.

The focus of the Clinton Foundation includes such concerns as improving global health, increasing opportunity for women and girls, reducing childhood obesity and preventable diseases, creating economic opportunity, and addressing issues of climate change. As a former president, Clinton continues to travel across the world, now focused mostly on activities of the Clinton Foundation.

Marian Wright Edelman (June 6, 1939–)

Marian Wright Edelman founded and was president of the Children's Defense Fund (CDF), a strong advocacy group for the rights and welfare of children and families. Under her leadership, CDF has become the nation's strongest voice for children and families. She graduated from Spelman College and Yale University Law School, and was the first African American woman admitted to the bar in Mississippi. She practiced law with the National Association for the Advancement of Colored People (NAACP) Legal Defense Fund and Educational Fund, and worked on issues linked to racial justice and the civil rights movement. In 1968, she moved to Washington, DC, where she continued her work on civil rights issues through Martin Luther King Jr.'s Poor People's campaign and with the Southern Christian Leadership Conference. After that, she joined the Washington Research Project, a public interest law firm, and her interests expanded from civil rights more generally to issues related to childhood development and children in general.

In 1973, she founded the Children's Defense Fund to be a voice for poor children, children of color, and children with other problems, such as disabilities. As the issues of poverty, education, and health (including access to healthcare) of America's children are strongly interrelated, Edelman and her advocacy group have been leading efforts to increase the government's efforts to support the welfare of this country's children. Her agency was a major public advocate for the passage of the CHIP (Child Health Insurance Program) legislation, which many viewed as the largest expansion of publicly funded healthcare since the passage of Medicare and Medicaid in 1965. This legislation has greatly reduced the number of uninsured children in the United States, although issues of adequate funding for the state-required match and enrollment of children may partially limit the success of this effort. Another effort by CDF has been to modify and increase the comprehensiveness of public welfare legislation. With major modifications, this effort recently culminated in the passage of the comprehensive child welfare legislation known as the Leave No Child Behind program, which relates mostly to education reform. The group supported the ACA.

Alain C. Enthoven (September 10, 1930–)

Alain C. Enthoven is an American economist who is considered the creator of the concept of managed competition, which has developed into healthcare's managed care approach. Managed care came to dominance in the 1990s and has continued to be an important concept for some aspects of healthcare delivery such as the Medicare Part C option. It is not as important an aspect of healthcare reform in the ACA as it was proposed to be in the failed Clinton healthcare reform initiatives or in some earlier reform efforts discussed in the Carter administration.

Enthoven started his public service in the 1960s as one of Robert McNamara's chief Whiz Kids in the Defense Department. He was a deputy assistant secretary of defense from 1961 to 1965, and from 1965 to 1969, he was assistant secretary of defense for systems analysis. Since 1973, he has held the Marriner S. Eccles Professorship of Public and Private Management at Stanford University. In 1977, he presented his Consumer Choice Health Plan to the Carter administration, which he built on the concepts of prepaid group practice plans developed in the 1930s and 1940s and on the health maintenance organization (HMO) strategy pushed in the early 1970s. The plan was based on what he called regulated competition. He then added to the concept design proposals to deal with such issues as financing, biased selection, market segmentation, information costs, and equity. The key to his vision of managed care is competition, with consumers having a choice among competing plans.

Across his career, he has published widely in the fields of the economics, organization, management, and public policy of healthcare in the United States, the United Kingdom, and the Netherlands. In addition to developing ideas related to managed competition, he has studied the causes of unsustainable growth in national health expenditures and the costs of health insurance, and he explored possible strategies for moderating this growth while improving quality of care. His later work has focused more on integrated delivery systems and on the potential for exchanges to correct some of the main deficiencies of employee-based health insurance. Many aspects of these approaches have been incorporated into the ACA.

Lyndon Baines Johnson (August 27, 1908–January 22, 1973)

After a long career in politics, first at the state level in Texas and then in the U.S. Senate, where he was the majority leader in the 1950s, Lyndon Baines Johnson (often known as LBJ) ran for vice president with John F. Kennedy on the ticket as president in 1960. Upon the assassination of President Kennedy in 1963, he became the thirty-sixth U.S. president. He was able to push the enactment of major civil rights and social legislation as part of his Great Society programs. A number of these programs were initially part of the Kennedy-Johnson platform for the 1960 election, but they were stalled in Congress and seemed unlikely to pass. Johnson was able to use the emotion of the Kennedy assassination, along with his excellent knowledge of Congress and how it worked, to get most of these programs put into place. His landslide election to the presidency on his own in 1964, which also swept into office larger Democratic majorities in Congress, made it easier to pass major legislation. Beyond the area health, much major social legislation dealing with education, welfare, and voting reform was passed.

The Johnson administration was responsible for the enactment of the two major U.S. government programs that still form the fundamental basis for the U.S. government's role in the direct provision of healthcare to Americans: Medicare and Medicaid. Passage of Medicare legislation provided health insurance across the United States for older adults and those with serious disabilities at a younger age. The coverage was comparable to that offered by many businesses at the time and was available to all Social Security recipients, independent of the amount of income and wealth they possessed. The Medicaid program provided healthcare coverage to recipients of major welfare programs through a joint federal-state program and thus was a benefit linked to a means-tested welfare system. This was part of an expansion of welfare-type benefits that were known as the Great Society initiative.

Despite his huge successes in his domestic policy agenda, the later years of LBJ's term in office were marred by the growth of the Vietnam War and the antiwar movement. There was so much protest that Johnson announced he would not run for another term, due to the dissension in the country. He retired to his ranch in Texas as a bystander to political activity, as his own vice president, Hubert Humphrey, was not able to win the 1968 election against Richard Nixon. LBJ became known as a tragic figure in American politics, one who had enormous domestic policy accomplishments but left office feeling rejected, with many of his policies no longer politically popular.

Edward M. Kennedy (February 22, 1932–August 25, 2009)

Edward "Ted" Kennedy was the youngest brother of John F. Kennedy (the thirty-fifth president of the United States) and Robert F. Kennedy (attorney general in John's cabinet and presidential contender when he was assassinated in 1968). He was elected to the U.S. Senate from Massachusetts in 1962 when his brother John resigned to run for the presidency. By the time of his death in 2009, he was serving in his ninth term and was the third most senior senator in the history of the Senate.

Throughout his time in the Senate, Kennedy was a leading Democrat on health-related issues, as well as a major backer of many other liberal reforms. He was one of the earlier opponents of the Vietnam War and an important spokesperson for many liberal causes. At one point, he seemed likely to become a presidential candidate, as in 1969, he became the youngest-ever majority whip in the U.S. Senate and an early front-runner for the Democratic presidential nomination. However, on

July 18, 1969, he accidentally drove his car off an unmarked bridge on Chappaquiddick Island, near Martha's Vineyard, Massachusetts. His companion in the car, 28-year-old Mary Jo Kopechne, drowned. This created a scandal and led to his removing himself from any presidential considerations. A judge later found Ted Kennedy guilty of leaving the scene of an accident. After recovering from this scandal, he focused on his career in the Senate, and the causes he championed included those in the area of health. He became a candidate for president in 1980, though Jimmy Carter ended up winning the nomination. He remained in the Senate and became one of the most respected senators by the time of his death, someone who could work across party lines on issues he valued deeply, and he was viewed as a leading advocate for liberal social positions. He was known as the lion of the Senate.

Starting in the early 1970s, Kennedy introduced legislation for the establishment of a national healthcare system, which was close to proposals President Nixon was developing when his efforts were ended by the Watergate crisis. In more recent years, he was a key senator in the passage of the Health Insurance Portability and Accountability Act of 1996, which made it easier for those who change or lose their jobs to keep their health insurance. During the Clinton administration, he was a major advocate of the Children's Health Act of 1997 (CHIP), which made health insurance far more widely available to children through age 18 in all 50 states. He was a leader in the effort to enact the Patient's Bill of Rights, which was designed to end the abuses of HMOs and managed care health plans and provide greater protection for patients and physicians when dealing with insurance companies. In a more behind the scenes manner, he worked with then-governor of Massachusetts Mitt Romney to help advocate for healthcare insurance reform in Massachusetts; the Massachusetts plan was a model for the ACA plan. Near the end of his life, he saw the inauguration of Barack Obama as president and the push to attain healthcare reform, but the ACA legislation did not pass in Congress until after his death.

Mitch McConnell (February 20, 1942–)

The senior Republican senator from Kentucky, Mitch McConnell served as the Senate minority leader and spearheaded the opposition by Senate Republicans to healthcare reform during the first term of Obama's presidency. He served as the Senate minority leader from January 3, 2007 until the beginning of the new Congressional session in 2015, when due to the success of the Republican party in the off term elections he became the Senate Majority leader. He is the longest serving U.S. senator in Kentucky history, the seventh-most senior senator currently, and the fourth most senior Republican member of the Senate. After completing his undergraduate education at the University of Louisville and his law degree at the University of Kentucky, he served briefly in the military and then began working in politics by interning for Senator John Sherman Cooper of Kentucky. After that, he was an assistant to Senator Marlo Cook and a deputy assistant attorney general under President Ford. He won his first elected position as the Jefferson Country judge executive in 1977 and was reelected in 1981. In 1984, he ran for the U.S. Senate against a two-term Democratic incumbent and won by a very thin margin.

In his early years in the U.S. Senate, he was known as a centrist but, over time, and similar to both the party overall and his state, he became more conservative and changed his position on some issues such as collective bargaining rights and minimum wage increases. In foreign policy, initially, he was a person presidents of both parties could count on when seeking foreign aid, but he has grown more concerned about foreign assistance. On domestic issues, he has been in favor of allowing the National Security Agency to monitor telephone and electronic communication of suspected terrorists without a warrant. He has been opposed to campaign finance reform. In healthcare, he introduced the Common Sense Medical Malpractice Reform Act of 2001. The bill would require that a healthcare liability action be initiated within two years; noneconomic damages may not exceed $250,000; and punitive damages may be awarded only in specified situations. Most importantly, he voted against the Patient Protection and Affordable Care Act (the ACA) in December 2009, and he voted against the Healthcare and Education Reconciliation Act of 2010. Throughout 2014, he continued to call for the full repeal of the ACA and argued that Kentucky should be allowed to keep the state's health insurance exchange.

Barack Obama (August 4, 1961–)

Barack Obama was elected the forty-fourth president of the United States in 2008 and was reelected in 2012. He is the first African American president of the United States. He was born in Honolulu, Hawaii, and graduated from Columbia University and Harvard University Law School. Before going to law school, he decided to gain some real-world experience in a different type of setting and worked as a community organizer in Chicago for a few years. After finishing law school and having been the editor of the *Harvard Law Review*, he decided to return to Chicago, where he worked as a civil rights lawyer and also taught constitutional law at the University of Chicago. He became involved in politics there and served three terms in the Illinois Senate from 1997 to 2004, including service on the Health and Human Services Committee. He also ran unsuccessfully for the U.S. House of Representatives in 2000.

In 2004, Obama became the Democratic nominee for the Senate from Illinois, after winning a primary in March of that year. He was asked to keynote the Democratic National Convention in July of that year and began to receive national attention based on his well-received keynote speech. He was successfully elected to the Senate in November. He began his presidential campaign in 2007 and competed with Hilary Rodham Clinton, defeating her in enough primaries to win first the nomination and then the election against John McCain. Only nine months after being elected president, he won the 2009 Nobel Peace Prize. He entered the presidency at a time of economic crisis, and his first focus as president was to sign into law economic stimulus legislation to deal with the 2008 recession: the American Recovery and Reinvestment Act of 2009 and the Tax Relief, Unemployment, and Insurance Reauthorization and Job Creation Act of 2010.

In health-related issues, his first legislation was the extension of the CHIP program, a leftover issue from the Bush administration. Then his efforts turned to healthcare reform, resulting in the passage of the Patient Protection and Affordable Care Act (ACA) of 2010, also sometimes called Obamacare. Obama was reelected to a second term as president in 2012, defeating Republican nominee Mitt Romney. Some of his second-term legislative efforts have included the promotion of domestic policies related to gun control in response to the shooting at Sandy Hook Elementary School as well as other violence across the country and full equality for lesbian, gay, and bisexual Americans, including a push by the administration to have courts strike down the Defense of Marriage Act of 1996. In foreign policy, after major reductions in the numbers of troops involved in the Iraq and Afghanistan wars in his first term, the growth and military gains made by the Islamic state in Iraq after the 2011 withdrawal of U.S. troops has led to renewed U.S. involvement in Iraq and bombing in Iraq and Syria.

Peter Orszag (December 16, 1968–)

Peter Orszag, an American economist, was President Obama's first director of the Office of Management and Budget and served until the summer of 2010. He was an influential figure in designing the Obama administration's strategy for healthcare reform and also played an important role in advising Congress on the topic. Before joining the Obama administration, Orszag led the Congressional Budget Office and also served as an economic advisor in the Clinton administration. He has also been a distinguished visiting fellow at the Council on Foreign Relations and served as a visiting columnist for the *New York Times* Op-Ed page. After leaving the Obama administration, he served as a vice chairman of corporate and investment banking, chairman of the Public Sector Group, and chairman of the Financial Strategy and Solutions Group at Citigroup.

While the director of the Congressional Budget Office (CBO) from January 2007 to November 2008, he often drew attention to the importance of rising healthcare costs in the government's long-term fiscal problems. While at the CBO, he added 20 health analysts to the 30 already employed there. Once he became head of the Office of Management and Budget (OMB) under Obama, he focused on the problems of weak growth and high unemployment. During his time as head of OMB, he also focused on healthcare reform and met with insurance executives and health experts. Health reform was made one of the Obama administration's top legislative priorities. When Orszag left his post, most objective analysts praised both his impartiality and his brilliance in the position, stating that he helped prevent an economic meltdown early in his term and helped set up recovery afterward.

Nancy Pelosi (March 26, 1940–)

The speaker of the House of Representatives, California Democrat Nancy Pelosi guided the passage of healthcare reform in the House. Her encouragement of a reconciliation strategy in 2010 was vital to the final passage of healthcare reform. She has been the representative in the U.S. Congress from the city of San Francisco for 23 years. She is a major

Democratic Party leader and is the first woman to lead a major political party in the House of Representatives. She served as the Democratic leader from 2003 to 2011 and previously served as House Democratic whip for one year. She served as speaker of the House from 2007 to 2011, the first woman in U.S. history to do so. Then she remained the Democratic leader for the House of Representatives in the 112th Congress, when the Democrats lost control of the House of Representatives.

Born in Baltimore, Maryland, Pelosi comes from a politically connected family. Her father, Thomas D'Alesandro Jr., was the mayor of Baltimore for 12 years, and before that, he represented Baltimore in Congress for five terms. Her brother also served as mayor of Baltimore. She married and moved to San Francisco, where her own political involvement began. She started in local Democratic politics and eventually became party chairwoman for northern California, serving as the head of the host committee for the Democratic National Convention in 1984. Pelosi won a special election to succeed Sala Burton, taking office on June 2, 1987. The next year (1988), she was elected to a full term and has easily held the seat since. Her district is safely Democratic, with only 13 percent of registered voters being Republican. Her safe seat has helped her be able to advance in the Democratic leadership in the House.

While speaker of the House, she helped pass a number of Obama's major initiatives such as health reform, the American Recovery and Reinvestment Act in early 2009, and Wall Street–related reforms. In addition, during her term as speaker, the extension of the State Child Health Insurance Plan (SCHIP) was passed, as was the Lilly Ledbetter Fair Pay Act, which is meant to help women fight pay discrimination. One of the major issues across her career has been energy security, and she was successful in helping pass comprehensive energy legislation in 2007 that raised vehicle fuel efficiency standards and included a commitment to American home-grown biofuels.

Ron Pollack (February 21, 1944–)

Ron Pollack is an attorney and activist on public policy issues. He is the director of Families USA, an advocacy group representing families. Prior to this position, he was the dean of the Antioch School of Law. During 1997–1998, Pollack was appointed to serve on the Presidential Advisory Commission on Consumer Protection and Quality in the Healthcare Industry. He was the sole representative from a consumer organization on that body. He worked on the preparation of the Patient's Bill of Rights, legislation to help improve the ability of patients to have options and to be able to register formal complaints against healthcare insurance companies, healthcare management companies, and other healthcare providers.

He is also the founder and chair of the Health Assistance Partnership, an entity that works with healthcare ombudsman programs across the country to help consumers navigate the increasingly complex U.S. healthcare system. Pollack is now also the founding board chairman of Enroll America, an organization that includes many diverse stakeholders who work together to secure optimal enrollment of uninsured people through effective implementation of the Affordable Care Act.

Although families are an important focus of the Families USA advocacy group, the organization has also focused on health issues since its inception as the Villers Foundation in 1982. His organization was one of the groups that pushed for passage of CHIP (Child Health Insurance Program) as a step forward in health insurance coverage for families, through the provision of health insurance coverage to children of the near poor and working poor. This legislation has been important in improving the rates of health insurance coverage for children under 18 years of age. The current mission of Families USA is to achieve high-quality, affordable health coverage for everyone in the United States. Families USA is an influential healthcare lobbyist in Washington, DC, and has taken positions on every major piece of healthcare legislation. In addition to lobbying and other efforts,

Pollack has expanded further the activities of Families USA as a partner with major nonprofit research groups. In 2013, Families USA received a $1 million grant from the Robert Wood Johnson Foundation to work together to publicize people's Affordable Care Act success stories.

Harry Reid (December 2, 1939–)

Harry Reid was first elected to the U.S. Senate representing Nevada in 1986 after representing Nevada's First Cong-ressional District from 1983 to 1987. He is now the senior sen-ator from Nevada. After attending college in Utah and law school in Washington, DC, he returned to Nevada and served as Henderson city attorney then was elected to the state assembly in 1968. In 1970, at the age of 30, he ran for lieuten-ant governor in Nevada and served in that post from 1971 until 1974. He then ran for a vacant Senate seat but lost by 700 votes to a former governor of the state, Paul Laxalt. He served as the chairman of the Nevada Gaming Commission from 1977 to 1981. Then his career first in the House of Representatives and then in the Senate began. Reid became Senate Demo-cratic minority whip in 2005, and he became Senate majority leader after the 2006 elections in which the Democrats success-fully regained control of the Senate.

As Senate majority leader, he was responsible for putting together healthcare legislation that could obtain the 60 votes needed to override a Republican filibuster. After several weeks of intense negotiations in December 2009, the Senate passed its version of healthcare reform. Reid faced a tough reelection battle in Nevada in 2010, where at one point, he trailed the two leading Republican candidates for his seat by about 10 per-cent. But he prevailed. During his time in Congress, Reed has sponsored a number of pieces of important legislation, includ-ing some linked to health. Reid helped obtain the passage of the Patient Protection and Affordable Care Act in the Senate.

He believes that *Roe vs. Wade* should be overturned and has voted against amendments that support Roe. He has also focused on immigration reform; one of his priorities has been passage of the Dream Act, which would allow certain high school graduates who are in the United States illegally to obtain conditional legal status so that they can serve in the military or attend college.

Kathleen Sebelius (May 15, 1948–)

Kathleen Sebelius was selected by president-elect Obama to be his first secretary of Health and Human Services, a key position given his agenda to pass major healthcare reform in his first year in office. Her previous political offices included time in the Kansas House of Representatives from 1985 to 1987. She left that position to run for state insurance commissioner in Kansas. She ran as a reform candidate who refused to take campaign contributions from the insurance industry. While in office, she blocked the proposed merger of Blue Cross–Blue Shield of Kansas with an Indiana-based company. She served as governor of Kansas from 2003 to 2009. Overall, she had a strong record as governor, being named by *Time* magazine as one of the five best governors in America in 2005. She reduced state debt, located and corrected waste in state government, and strongly supported public education. She was reelected to a second term, which was more difficult. Fights over tax revenue led to spending cuts in the state, including in education, an area of great importance to her. During the 2004 election, some had speculated she could be John Kerry's running mate in his bid for president, but she was not chosen. Some also mentioned her as a possible candidate for president in 2008. There was speculation she might be the vice presidential candidate with Obama, but this did not happen. Nor was she initially offered a cabinet post, despite some speculation that she might become the secretary of commerce. After Tom Daschle was forced to withdraw as Obama's nominee for secretary of health and human services due to tax problems, her name was discussed as a replacement, and she did become Obama's first secretary of health and human services.

Sebelius worked hard for the passage of the Affordable Care Act and then for its implementation. When the enrollment website started to experience problems, she apologized for its failures. Republicans called for her resignation, which did not happen at that time, but the problems began to overall negatively impact her position. In April 2014, after the first enrollment period through the exchanges for the ACA was completed, she announced her resignation, ending a long and mostly successful career in politics. While none of the enrollment website problems were her own personal failures, as the secretary of health and human services, criticism focused on her, and she was willing to be replaced to try and give a new person a fresh start at improvement for the rest of the year and the second open enrollment period.

Government Agencies

The government agencies that are most involved in the healthcare system are also key sources for relevant data used in researching healthcare and its reform and are described in Chapter 5, "Data and Documents." This chapter presents information on two additional key government agencies that significantly impact healthcare reform.

Congressional Budget Office

The Congressional Budget Office (http://www.cbo.gov/) was set up in 1974 to produce independent analyses of budgetary and economic issues to support the congressional budget process. The agency is strictly nonpartisan and conducts objective, impartial analysis, which is evident in each of the dozens of reports and hundreds of cost estimates that its economists and policy analysts produce each year. It plays a major role in the health reform legislative process with its reports on the financial impact of different proposed health reform–related legislation. It also has produced reports on Medicare, Medicaid, CHIP, the Affordable Care Act, private health insurance, public health, and prevention. Recent reports related to health reform published by the CBO include:

An Update to the Budget and Economic Outlook: 2014 to 2024 (http://www.cbo.gov/publication/45653, October 2014). Report August 27, 2014. The deficit this year will be $506 billion, CBO estimates, about $170 billion lower than the deficit in 2013. After a weak first half of this year, CBO expects economic growth to pick up and the unemployment rate to continue to fall.

Competition and the Cost of Medicare's Prescription Drug Program (http://www.cbo.gov/publication/45552, October 2014). Report July 30, 2014. Why has Medicare's prescription drug program cost less than anticipated when the program was created? How has competition between plan sponsors affected spending? How do Medicare Part D drug prices compare to those in Medicaid?

The 2014 Long-Term Budget Outlook (http://www.cbo .gov/publication/45471). Report July 15, 2014. If current laws remained generally unchanged, federal debt held by the public would exceed 100 percent of GDP by 2039 and would be on an upward path relative to the size of the economy—a trend that could not be sustained indefinitely.

Updated Estimates of the Effects of the Insurance Coverage Provisions of the Affordable Care Act, April 2014 (http://www.cbo.gov/publication/45231, October 2014). Report April 14, 2014. CBO and JCT have lowered their estimates of the net federal cost of the ACA's insurance coverage provisions—to $1.4 trillion over the next decade, about $100 billion less than estimated in February.

U.S. Supreme Court

The U.S. Supreme Court provided the final ruling on the constitutionality of the Affordable Care Act. In June 2012, it ruled that the act is constitutional, with the deciding vote in a 5–4 split made by Chief Justice John G. Roberts Jr. This and other cases relating to health reform moving through the courts for probable review by the Supreme Court are discussed in Chapter 2.

Organizations and Think Tanks

Chapters 5 and 6 provide a good overview of the types of organizations with a significant focus on health reform and the types of information they make available. This section highlights several additional organizations in more detail as a further example of the diverse interests and organizations involved in the healthcare debate.

Families USA

Families USA (http://www.familiesusa.org) is a progressive advocacy group whose work with the Clinton and Obama administrations' efforts passing health reform has led "to the achievement of high-quality, affordable health and long-term care for all Americans." It was founded in 1981 under the name Villers Foundation by cofounders Ron Pollack (who currently serves as the group's executive director and vice president) and Philippe Villers, who is currently the organization's president. In 1997, President Bill Clinton appointed Pollack as the sole consumer representative on the Presidential Advisory Commission on Consumer Protection and Quality in the Healthcare Industry, where he worked on the Patient's Bill of Rights.

Villers serves on the American Civil Liberty Union's (ACLU) President's Committee and Amnesty International USA's Executive Directors Council. The organization strongly supported passage of the Affordable Care Act and is trying to assist people eligible for healthcare coverage under ACA to enroll. Its Research and Publications page provides links to reports and infographics.

National Association of Community Health Centers (NACHC)

The National Association of Community Health Centers was organized in 1971 to work with a network of state health center and primary care organizations to serve health centers in a variety of ways:

- Provide research-based advocacy for health centers and their clients
- Educate the public about the mission and value of health centers
- Train and provide technical assistance to health center staff and boards
- Develop alliances with private partners and key stakeholders to foster the delivery of primary healthcare services to communities in need

There are almost 1,300 health centers operating at over 9,200 service delivery sites that provide care to more than 21.7 million patients in every U.S. state, the District of Columbia, Puerto Rico, the U.S. Virgin Islands, and the Pacific basin. One out of 15 people currently living in the United States receives primary healthcare from a community health center.

The Affordable Care Act established the Community Health Center Fund, which provides $11 billion over a five-year period for the operation, expansion, and construction of health centers throughout the nation. The Health Resources and Services Administration (HRSA) states in its fact sheet titled *The Affordable Care Act and Health Centers*:

> Health centers are poised to play an essential role in the implementation of the Affordable Care Act. In particular, health centers emphasize coordinated primary and preventive services or a "medical home" that promotes reductions in health disparities for low–income individuals, racial and ethnic minorities, rural communities and other underserved populations. Health centers place emphasis on the co-ordination and comprehensiveness of care, the ability to manage patients with multiple healthcare needs, and the use of key quality improvement practices, including health information technology. The health center model also over-comes geographic, cultural, linguistic and other barriers through a team–based approach to care that includes physi-cians, nurse practitioners, physician assistants, nurses, dental providers, midwives, behavioral healthcare providers, social workers, health educators, and many others. (http://bphc .hrsa.gov/about/healthcenterfactsheet.pdf)

National Federation of Independent Business (NFIB)

The National Federation of Independent Business (http:// www.nfib.com/) is the largest small business association representing small and independent businesses in the United States. It provides group purchasing power for its members and advocates on issues of importance to small business. While originally supporting health reform, NFIB opposed the final health reform legislation signed into to law by President Obama as being too expensive for small businesses. Its health policy page (http://www.nfib.com/foundations/research-foundation/ studies/health-policy/) presents the following sections which link to the group's policies and supporting documents:

Understanding the New Healthcare Law (http://www
.nfib.com/article/understanding-the-new-healthcare-law-
51298/). The new healthcare legislation was signed into
law March 23, 2010, leaving many small business owners
wondering: What does this mean for me? What do I have
to do now? NFIB has answers.

**The Healthcare Playbook: A Small Business Guide to
PPACA** (http://www.nfib.com/Portals/0/PDF/AllUsers/
advocacy/ppaca-healthcare-law-guide-nfib.pdf). This print-
able document provides details about the time line of new
fees and regulations set to take effect, as well as information
about whether these provisions will affect you and your
business.

Rand Corporation

Rand Corporation (http://www.rand.org/) is a major public
policy–oriented research institute that began during World
War II and since then has become an independent nonprofit
research and policy organization. With a staff of 1,700 (of
whom about 1,000 are research staff), Rand conducts research
on a wide variety of public policy topics, including healthcare,
education, and welfare. Rand's 2013 funding of over
$63 million came from a number of sources, the largest of
which was state, local, and national government grants and
projects. Rand also operates the Pardee Rand Graduate School,
which, with about 100 PhD students, is the world's leading
producer of doctorate-level public policy analysts. Health and
healthcare is a focus area of Rand's research. The health and
healthcare area page on the organization's website provides links
to numerous full-text reports and briefs related to "innovative
studies of health insurance, healthcare reform, health information
technology, and women's health, as well as topical concerns such
as obesity, complementary and alternative medicine, and PTSD
in veterans and survivors of catastrophe."

Tea Party Movement

The Tea Party movement is a loosely defined, ultraconservative, populist antitax movement that arose in 2009 in a series of protests in reaction to the Obama presidency and the health-care reform debate. The initial impetus came from opposition to the administration's stimulus package, the American Recovery and Reinvestment Act of 2009. Most of its efforts in 2010 focused on strong opposition to health reform legislation. Its tactics were often aggressive and disruptive, as it modeled its actions on those of radical left movements of the 1960s and 1970s. Tea Party movement participants are united in their opposition to President Obama's perceived high tax liberal agenda in general, and his healthcare reform program specifically. However, the movement has not been able to form a broad agenda that can pull the membership together into a more long-term movement or party. In 2010, the movement helped elect very conservative right-wing candidates to the U.S. House of Representatives. This solidified the far right wing of the party, making it harder for the Republican caucus to work with the Democratic side of the House and with the Democratically controlled Senate. In 2012, the movement was unsuccessful in its attempts to defeat President Obama's reelection bid. Since that election, the split in the Republican Party between the hard right and the traditional pro-business fiscally conservative factions has widened. In the contentious Republican primaries leading to the 2014 mid-term election, the traditional side of the party won every primary except for the surprising loss of Eric Cantor, the second-highest leader in the Republican House caucus. The Tea Party is named in reference to the 1773 Boston Tea Party, which was protesting British taxation policies. Several groups claim to represent the movement, including:

- Tea Party Patriots: http://teapartypatriots.ning.com/; healthcare page at http://www.teapartypatriots.org/all-issues/issues/healthcare/

- Tea Party Nation: http://www.teapartynation.com/
- Tea Party Express: http://www.teapartyexpress.org/
- Tea Party: http:// http://www.teaparty.org/

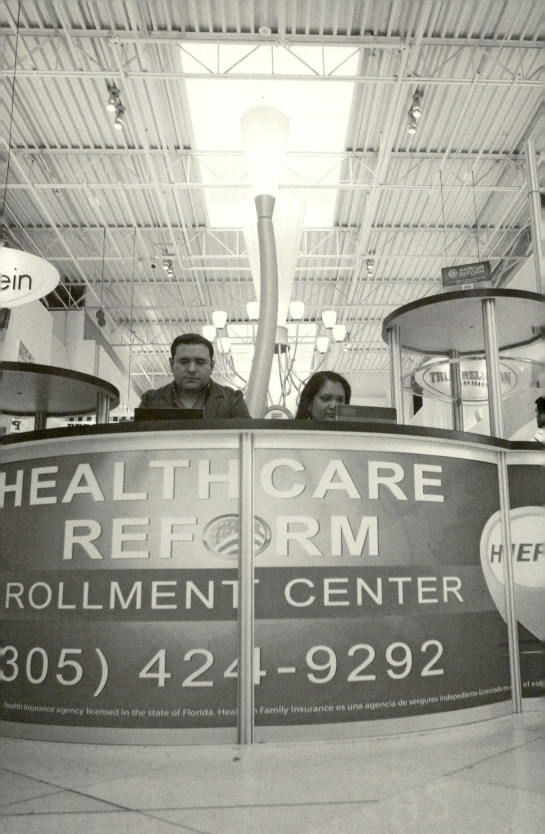

HEALTH CARE
REF☉RM
ROLLMENT CENTER
305) 424-9292

H ER

health insurance agency licensed in the state of Florida. Health Family Insurance es una agencia de serguros indepediente licenciada en el est

Much of the data available in healthcare are collected at the federal level and are readily available via federal agency websites. Data on specific states is also available through the federal government's websites; in addition, some state agencies have state and local data available. There is also a centralized website, htpp:// www.fedstats.gov, that provides easy access to government information sorted by topics. One of the topics is health.

Government Data Sources

While there are many different federal agencies that have some information related to health, the four most relevant are AHRQ (Agency for Health Care Research and Quality), CMS (Centers for Medicare and Medicaid Services), HRSA (Health Resources and Services Administration), and the National Center for Health Statistics (NCHS) at the Centers for Disease Control and Prevention (CDC).

National Center for Health Statistics (NCHS)

Of the four major federal agencies that collect health-related data, the most important, and the one containing the most

---

Jorge Espinoa and Cristian Hernandez man a healthcare reform booth at the Dolphin Mall in Sweetwater, Florida on November 28, 2014 as shoppers pass by. The pair working for Health Family Insurance said that a few people had stopped by. (AP Photo/J Pat Carter)

data, is the National Center for Health Statistics (NCHS) (http://www.cdc.gov/nchs/), which is part of the Centers for Disease Control and Prevention (CDC). This agency is responsible for the collection, analysis, and dissemination of statistics on the nature and extent of the health, illness, and disability of the U.S. population. Its website collects statistics to:

- Document the health status of the population and of important subgroups
- Identify disparities in health status and use of healthcare by race or ethnicity, socioeconomic status, region, and other population characteristics
- Describe experiences with the healthcare system
- Monitor trends in health status and healthcare delivery
- Identify health problems
- Support biomedical and health services research
- Provide information for making changes in public policies and programs
- Evaluate the impact of health policies and programs

The **Centers for Disease Control and Prevention (CDC)** (http://www.cdc.gov/), headquartered in Atlanta, Georgia, is the component of NIH charged with direct protection of the public's health. Its mission is to:

> to protect America from health, safety and security threats, both foreign and in the U.S. Whether diseases start at home or abroad, are chronic or acute, curable or preventable, human error or deliberate attack, CDC fights disease and supports communities and citizens to do the same.

It accomplishes this through a focus on disease prevention and control (especially infectious diseases), environmental health, occupational safety and health, health promotion, prevention, and education activities. It provides data on:

- Morbidity
- Infectious and chronic diseases
- Occupational diseases and injuries
- Vaccine efficacy and safety studies

Some examples of the more specific topics on which data is gathered by this agency include information on:

- The common cold
- Influenza, including H1N1
- Asthma
- Diabetes
- Disabilities and impairments
- Health insurance coverage
- Heart disease
- Home health and hospice care
- Hospital utilization
- Hypertension
- Child and infant health
- Mammography and breast cancer
- Men's health.

NCHS aggregates data to provide information about the key national indicators of well-being, the leading causes of death, and typical life expectancy figures for various population groups. These types of data are important in determining how well a country's healthcare system is functioning and whether there are important groups within the country (based on geographical criteria, race and ethnicity, or other factors) that are not having a positive experience in their overall health and health-care. The CDC's Data and Statistics page (http://www.cdc.gov/DataStatistics/) is the best site to begin searching for CDC data.

Agency for Healthcare Research and Quality (AHRQ)

AHRQ (http://www.ahrq.gov/) is the health services research component of the Department of Health and Human Services (DHHS), complementing the National Institutes of Health (NIH), which is the biomedical branch of the agency. Its research centers focus on:

- Quality improvement and patient safety
- Outcomes and effectiveness of care
- Clinical practice and technology assessment
- Healthcare organization and delivery systems
- Primary care (including preventive services)
- Healthcare costs and sources of payment

The organization produces and disseminates scientific and policy-relevant information about the cost, quality, access, and medical effectiveness of healthcare. AHQR maintains several databases, including the following:

The **Medical Expenditure Panel Survey (MEPS)** (http://meps.ahrq.gov/mepsweb), is the most complete source of data on the cost and use of healthcare and health insurance coverage.

The **Healthcare Cost & Utilization Project** (HCUP) (http://www.hcup-us.ahrq.gov/) is a family of healthcare databases and related software tools and products developed through a federal-state-industry partnership and sponsored by the Agency for Healthcare Research and Quality (AHRQ). HCUP databases include:

- The Kids' Inpatient Database (KID) is a nationwide sample of pediatric inpatient discharges.
- The Nationwide Emergency Department Sample (NEDS) is a database that yields national estimates of emergency department (ED) visits.
- The State Inpatient Databases (SID) contain the universe of inpatient discharge abstracts from participating states.
- The State Ambulatory Surgery Databases (SASD) contain data from ambulatory care encounters from hospital-affiliated and sometimes freestanding ambulatory surgery sites.
- The State Emergency Department Databases (SEDD) contain data from hospital-affiliated emergency departments for visits that do not result in hospitalizations.

Centers for Medicare and Medicaid Services

CMS (http://cms.hhs.gov/) is responsible for the operation and administration of the Medicare program and works with state governments to administer the Medicaid, State Child Health Insurance Program (SCHIP), and Health Insurance Marketplace programs. Its goal is to administer these programs in an effective and efficient manner to provide quality healthcare to the nation's poor and older adults with a minimum of fraud and waste. In doing so, it collects administrative data associated with its oversight of Medicare and Medicaid, and also studies the quality of care delivered by those programs. The CMS website is rich in statistics and reports relating to the programs it administers and coordinates, which provide health coverage for over 100 million Americans.

- The **National Health Insurance Data** site (https://www.cms.gov/Research-Statistics-Data-and-Systems/Statistics-Trends-and-Reports/NationalHealthExpendData/index.html) contains data and analysis of recent trends in healthcare spending, employment, and prices.
- The **CMS Data Navigator** (http://dnav.cms.gov/) is a menu-driven search tool that makes the data and information resources of the Centers for Medicare and Medicaid Services (CMS) more easily available.

- The **Research, Statistics, Data & Systems** site (https:// www.cms.gov/Research-Statistics-Data-and-Systems/Research -Statistics-Data-and-Systems.html) and the **Active Reports** site (http://www.cms.gov/Research-Statistics-Data-and-Systems/ Statistics-Trends-and-Reports/ActiveProjectReports/index. html?redirect=/ActiveProjectReports/APR/list.asp#TopOfPage) list active CMS research projects for the year of the annual report.

Health Resources and Services Administration (HRSA)

HRSA (http://www.hrsa.gov/) is the primary federal agency for improving access to healthcare services for people who are uninsured, isolated, or medically vulnerable. HRSA funds healthcare and medications for about half of the people in the United States with HIV/AIDS. It oversees all organ, bone marrow, and cord blood donations programs and monitors trends in the healthcare workforce. In carrying out its duties, it collects data about general health services, the health professions workforce, and resource issues relating to access, equity, quality, and cost of care. It also maintains the Scientific Registry for organ transplants. Its major data resources are:

- The **United States Health Professions** site (http://bhpr.hrsa .gov/healthworkforce/). This site provides Area Health Resources Files (AHRF), which include basic county, state, and national files. These files provide a comprehensive set of data that offers a broad range of health resources and socioeconomic indicators that impact demand for healthcare. Data is current and historic for more than 6,000 variables for each of the nation's counties. The site also contains data on health facilities, compiled from more than a dozen professional associations and government agencies.
- The **Data Warehouse** site (http://datawarehouse.hrsa .gov/) allows users to manipulate data through charts, maps, reports, analyzer and locator tools, data downloads and data services, and widgets.

HRSA is a good place to begin searching for data relevant to understanding the healthcare system and its reform.

Other Federal Agencies

Some of the other federal agencies that provide specialized health-related data are discussed in this section.

The **Indian Health Service (IHS)** (http://www.ihs.gov/) is the primary healthcare provider and advocate for American Indians and Alaska Natives. It collects social and economic statistics, as well as patient care and morbidity information for those who use IHS services.

The **National Institutes of Health (NIH)** (http://www.nih.gov/) is the primary federal agency supporting research in clinical medicine. Within 27 institutes and centers, the NIH supports the investigation of ways to prevent disease as well as the causes, treatments, and even cures for common and rare diseases. It supports the design and implementation of epidemiological studies, clinical trials, biomedical research, and laboratory investigations conducted by the various institutes. The following institutes have set up specific websites with statistics in the area of their focus:

- Cancer: http://www.nci.nih.gov/statistics/
- Deafness and Other Communication Disorders: http://www.nidcd.nih.gov/health/statistics/Pages/Default.aspx
- Dental Health: http://www.nidcr.nih.gov/DataStatistics/
- Diabetes and Digestive and Kidney Diseases: http://www.niddk.nih.gov/health-information/health-statistics/Pages/default.aspx
- Drug Abuse: http://www.nida.nih.gov/DrugPages/Stats.html
- Eye Health: http://www.nida.nih.gov/DrugPages/Stats.html
- Mental Health: http://www.nimh.nih.gov/health/topics/statistics/index.shtml

The **Substance Abuse and Mental Health Services Administration (SAMHSA)** (http://www.samhsa.gov/) provides information on health problems related to the use and abuse of drugs and alcohol, substance abuse treatment, and the mental health condition of the population. It administers and evaluates federal block grants to the states. Its Data, Outcomes, and Quality site (http://www.samhsa.gov/data/) presents links to surveys and data collection systems, publications, and data files.

Historical Health Data

The best sources for historical data are two government publications—*Statistical Abstract of the United States*, published annually by the U.S. Census Bureau, and *Health, United States*, published annually by NCHS.

The *Statistical Abstract of the United States* (http://www .census.gov/compendia/statab/) is the national data book for the United States and contains a collection of statistics on social and economic conditions in the United States. One of its major sections is Health and Nutrition (http://www.census .gov/compendia/statab/cats/health_nutrition.html). This section presents tables with data by year, with some tables going back as far as 1960 and with many going back as far as 1990. The site provides online access to the abstracts back to 1887 along with vital statistics and health data back to the colonial period.

Health, United States (http://www.cdc.gov/nchs/hus.htm) is an annual report on national trends in health statistics. Published annually, it provides data in tables on 24 topics relating to healthcare in the United States. The topics in the 2013 edition are:

- American Indian or Alaska Native population
- Asian or Pacific Islander population
- Black or African American population
- Child and adolescent health
- Disability
- Diseases and conditions
- Education

- Health expenditures
- Health insurance
- Health risk factors
- Hispanic or Latino population
- Infectious disease
- Injury
- Men's health
- Mental health
- Metropolitan and nonmetropolitan areas
- Older population
- Poverty
- Preventive care
- Special feature: prescription drugs
- State data
- White population
- Women's health
- Working-age adults

Many of the tables go back 20 years or more. The annual editions on the website are available back to 1975.

Data and Documents from Government Sources

The following charts display how the nation's dollars were used for healthcare in 2012. Figure 5.1 shows where the money within the healthcare system comes from. Figure 5.2 displays how the nation's healthcare dollars are spent.

The following tables are but a sampling of the wealth of data presented in two key federal documents describes earlier in this chapter, *The Statistical Abstract of the United States* and *Health, United States*. The tables are from the 2012 editions (the most recent available at publication); new editions are published on the Internet every year.

The Nation's Health Dollar ($2.8 Trillion), Calendar Year 2012: Where It Came From

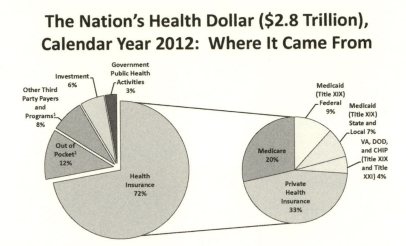

[1] Includes worksite health care, other private revenues, Indian Health Service, workers' compensation, general assistance, maternal and child health, vocational rehabilitation, Substance Abuse and Mental Health Services Administration, school health, and other federal and state local programs.
[2] Includes co-payments, deductibles, and any amounts not covered by health insurance.
Note: Sum of pieces may not equal 100% due to rounding.

SOURCE: Centers for Medicare & Medicaid Services, Office of the Actuary, National Health Statistics Group.

Figure 5.1   The Nation's Health Dollar ($2.8 Trillion), Calendar Year 2012: Where It Came From

Source: http://www.cms.gov/Research-Statistics-Data-and-Systems/Statistics-Trends-and-Reports/NationalHealthExpendData/Downloads/PieChartSourcesExpenditures2012.pdf.

Table 5.1 presents extensive data on national health expenditures from 1960 to 2009. Several observations can be made from this table. One is the absolute increase in expenditures, with a 91-fold increase in the 49 years from 1960 to 2009. Hospital care and physician and clinical services represent 61 percent of total expenditures for personal healthcare. The next highest category is prescription drugs, representing 12 percent.

Table 5.2 focuses on the source of funds from 1990 to 2009. It provides the annual percentage change, the percentage of gross domestic product represented by health expenditures that specific year, and more details on the sources of expenditures, both private and public.

Table 5.3 provides data about hospital care, physician and clinical services, nursing care facilities and continuing care

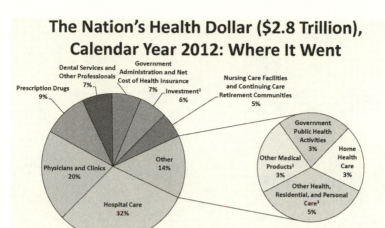

The Nation's Health Dollar ($2.8 Trillion), Calendar Year 2012: Where It Went

[1] Includes Non-commercial Research (2%) and Structures and Equipment (4%).
[2] Includes Durable (1%) and Non-durable (2%) goods.
[3] Includes expenditures for residential care facilities, ambulance providers, medical care delivered in non-traditional settings (such as community centers, senior citizens centers, schools, and military field stations), and expenditures for Home and Community Waiver programs under Medicaid.
Note: Sum of pieces may not equal 100% due to rounding.

SOURCE: Centers for Medicare & Medicaid Services, Office of the Actuary, National Health Statistics Group.

Figure 5.2 The Nation's Health Dollar ($2.8 Trillion), Calendar Year 2012: Where It Went

Source: http://www.cms.gov/Research-Statistics-Data-and-Systems/Statistics-Trends-and-Reports/NationalHealthExpendData/Downloads/PieChartSourcesExpenditures2012.pdf.

retirement communities, and prescription drug expenditures from 1990 to 2009. Of particular interest is the comparison between out of pocket and public and private insurance sources.

Table 5.4 provides information about average annual expenditures per consumer unit, providing figures for 2007 through 2009. The figures are also categorized by certain basic characteristics of the person, such as age, race, origin, size of consumer unit, and income. Depending on the interest of the reader, this table provides a great deal of information about variation in expenditures. Looking at the age figures, the amount column makes the point clearly that average annual expenditures increase as people become older. The table also illustrates that this trend of increasing expenditures by age is true for health insurance and drugs and medical supplies

Table 5.1. National Health Expenditures—Summary: 1960 to 2009

(In billions of dollars [27.3 represents $27,300,000,000]. Excludes Puerto Rico and Island Areas)

Year	National health expenditures, total[1]	Health consumption expenditures, total[2]	Personal healthcare expenditures										
			Total[3]	Hospital care	Physician and clinical services	Other professional services	Dental services	Other health residential and personal care	Home healthcare	Nursing care facilities[4]	Prescription drugs	Durable medical equipment	Other non-durable medical equipment
1960	27.3	24.8	23.3	9.0	5.6	0.4	2.0	0.5	0.1	0.8	2.7	0.7	1.6
1961	29.2	26.3	24.8	9.8	5.8	0.4	2.1	0.5	0.1	0.8	2.7	0.8	1.8
1962	31.9	28.4	26.6	10.4	6.3	0.4	2.2	0.6	0.1	0.9	3.0	0.9	1.9
1963	34.7	30.9	29.0	11.5	7.1	0.5	2.3	0.6	0.1	1.0	3.2	0.9	1.9
1964	38.5	34.1	32.0	12.5	8.1	0.5	2.6	0.7	0.1	1.2	3.3	1.0	2.1
1965	41.9	37.2	34.7	13.5	8.6	0.5	2.8	0.7	0.1	1.4	3.7	1.1	2.2
1966	46.2	41.2	38.4	15.3	9.3	0.6	3.0	0.8	0.1	1.7	4.0	1.2	2.4
1967	51.7	46.5	43.5	17.8	10.4	0.6	3.4	0.9	0.1	2.2	4.2	1.1	2.5
1968	58.7	52.7	49.2	20.5	11.4	0.6	3.7	1.1	0.2	2.9	4.7	1.3	2.8
1969	66.2	59.1	55.5	23.4	12.7	0.7	4.2	1.2	0.2	3.4	5.1	1.5	3.0
1970	74.8	67.0	63.1	27.2	14.3	0.7	4.7	1.3	0.3	4.0	5.5	1.7	3.3
1971	83.2	74.3	69.4	30.2	15.9	0.8	5.2	1.4	0.2	4.6	5.9	1.8	3.5
1972	93.1	83.3	77.1	33.8	17.7	0.9	5.5	1.7	0.2	5.2	6.3	2.0	3.7
1973	103.3	93.1	86.1	37.9	19.6	1.0	6.3	2.0	0.3	6.0	6.8	2.2	4.0
1974	117.1	105.9	98.8	44.1	22.2	1.2	7.1	2.4	0.4	6.9	7.4	2.5	4.5
1975	133.5	121.1	113.2	51.2	25.3	1.3	8.0	2.9	0.6	8.0	8.1	2.8	4.9
1976	153.0	139.3	129.3	59.4	28.7	1.6	9.0	3.6	0.9	9.1	8.7	3.0	5.4

Year													
1977	173.9	159.9	146.7	67.0	33.1	2.1	10.1	4.5	1.1	10.3	9.2	3.2	6.1
1978	195.4	180.0	164.3	75.6	35.8	2.4	11.0	5.6	1.6	11.8	9.9	3.4	7.1
1979	221.6	204.6	187.2	86.2	41.2	2.8	11.9	6.8	1.9	13.3	10.7	3.8	8.5
1980	255.7	235.6	217.1	100.5	47.7	3.5	13.3	8.5	2.4	15.3	12.0	4.1	9.8
1981	296.6	273.5	251.9	117.5	55.6	4.3	15.7	9.6	2.9	17.3	13.4	4.3	11.3
1982	334.6	308.2	283.2	133.6	61.6	4.9	17.0	10.9	3.5	19.5	15.0	4.6	12.6
1983	368.8	339.6	311.8	144.7	68.7	5.7	18.3	12.2	4.2	21.7	17.3	5.3	13.8
1984	406.3	375.3	341.9	154.4	77.4	7.3	19.8	13.3	5.1	23.7	19.6	6.1	15.0
1985	444.4	413.2	376.8	164.6	90.8	8.1	21.7	14.8	5.6	26.3	21.8	7.1	16.0
1986	476.7	444.2	409.4	175.7	100.7	9.3	23.1	16.0	6.4	28.7	24.3	8.1	17.1
1987	518.9	482.9	448.3	189.5	112.9	11.4	25.3	17.2	6.7	30.7	26.9	9.5	18.3
1988	581.5	541.3	499.3	206.5	128.6	13.8	27.3	19.2	8.4	34.3	30.6	11.1	19.4
1989	647.2	603.2	551.4	226.0	143.3	14.6	29.3	21.9	10.2	38.7	34.8	11.9	20.8
1990	724.0	675.3	616.6	250.4	158.9	17.4	31.5	24.3	12.6	44.9	40.3	13.8	22.4
1991	791.2	739.2	677.4	275.8	176.5	18.7	33.3	27.8	15.2	49.4	44.4	13.1	23.2
1992	857.7	800.8	733.4	298.5	191.3	21.0	37.0	30.1	18.7	53.1	47.0	13.5	23.2
1993	921.3	860.1	781.0	315.7	202.8	23.2	38.9	34.1	22.8	56.0	49.6	14.1	23.7
1994	972.5	908.6	823.0	328.4	212.2	24.2	41.5	38.1	27.4	58.6	53.1	15.3	24.3
1995	1,027.3	961.4	872.7	339.3	222.3	27.0	44.5	42.1	32.4	64.5	59.8	15.9	25.1
1996	1,081.6	1,013.9	921.7	350.8	231.3	29.2	46.8	46.6	35.8	69.6	68.1	17.4	26.0
1997	1,142.4	1,070.2	974.5	363.4	242.9	31.7	50.2	50.5	37.0	74.4	77.6	19.2	27.6
1998	1,208.6	1,128.5	1,028.3	374.9	257.9	33.8	53.5	56.2	34.2	79.4	88.4	21.3	28.6
1999	1,286.8	1,200.0	1,088.8	393.6	271.1	35.0	57.2	59.8	32.9	80.8	104.7	23.0	30.6
2000	1,378.0	1,288.5	1,164.4	415.5	290.0	37.0	62.0	64.7	32.4	85.1	120.9	25.1	31.6

(continued)

211

Table 5.1. (continued)

								Personal healthcare expenditures					
Year	National health expenditures, total[1]	Health consumption expenditures, total[2]	Total[3]	Hospital care	Physician and clinical services	Other professional services	Dental services	Other health residential and personal care	Home healthcare	Nursing care facilities[4]	Prescription drugs	Durable medical equipment	Other non-durable medical equipment
2001	1,495.3	1,401.4	1,264.1	449.4	314.7	40.6	67.5	70.7	34.4	90.8	138.7	25.1	32.3
2002	1,637.0	1,531.6	1,371.6	486.5	340.8	43.7	73.4	77.7	36.6	94.5	158.2	27.0	33.3
2003	1,772.2	1,658.2	1,479.0	525.8	368.4	46.8	76.0	84.0	39.8	100.1	175.2	27.8	35.1
2004	1,894.7	1,772.9	1,585.0	564.5	393.6	50.1	81.8	90.7	43.8	105.4	190.3	28.9	35.8
2005	2,021.0	1,890.3	1,692.6	606.5	419.6	53.1	86.8	96.5	48.7	112.1	201.7	30.4	37.2
2006	2,152.1	2,016.9	1,798.8	648.3	441.6	55.4	91.4	102.1	52.6	117.0	219.8	31.9	38.7
2007	2,283.5	2,135.1	1,904.3	686.8	462.6	59.5	97.3	108.3	57.8	126.5	230.2	34.4	41.1
2008	2,391.4	2,234.2	1,997.2	722.1	486.5	63.4	102.3	113.3	62.1	132.8	237.2	35.1	42.3
2009	2,486.3	2,330.1	2,089.9	759.1	505.9	66.8	102.2	122.6	68.3	137.0	249.9	34.9	43.3

[1]Includes Health Consumption Expenditures plus medical research, and medical structures and equipment.
[2]Includes Personal Health Expenditures plus government administration, net cost of health insurance, and government public health activities.
[3]Includes hospital care, physician and clinical services, dental services, other professional services, other health, residential, and personal services, home healthcare, nursing care facilities and continuing care retirement communities, prescription drugs, durable medical equipment, and other nondurable medical products.
[4]Includes care provided in nursing care facilities (NAICS 6231), continuing care retirement communities (623311), state and local government nursing facilities, and nursing facilities operated by the Department of Veterans' Affairs (DVA).
Source: U.S. Centers for Medicare and Medicaid Services, Office of the Actuary, "National Health Statistics Group."
For more information:
http://www.cms.gov/NationalHealthExpendData/
Internet release date: 09\30\2011
Source: http://www.census.gov/compendia/statab/2012/tables/12s0134.pdf.

212

Table 5.2a. National Health Expenditures by Source of Funds: 1990 to 1999

(In billions of dollars [724.0 represents $724,000,000,000], except percent. Excludes Puerto Rico and Island Areas.)

Source of Funds	1990	1991	1992	1993	1994	1995	1996	1997	1998	1999
National health expenditure, total	**724.0**	**791.2**	**857.7**	**921.3**	**972.5**	**1,027.3**	**1,081.6**	**1,142.4**	**1,208.6**	**1,286.8**
Annual percent change[1]	11.9	9.3	8.4	7.4	5.6	5.6	5.3	5.6	5.8	6.5
Percent of gross domestic product	12.5	13.2	13.5	13.8	13.7	13.9	13.8	13.7	13.7	13.8
Out-of-pocket	**138.8**	**141.8**	**144.3**	**145.4**	**143.5**	**146.4**	**152.9**	**164.6**	**180.0**	**190.7**
Health insurance	**439.2**	**492.6**	**543.8**	**594.1**	**638.0**	**682.9**	**723.5**	**760.4**	**794.0**	**847.1**
Private health insurance	233.9	255.3	275.4	296.2	309.4	326.8	345.1	361.7	386.8	419.0
Medicare	110.2	120.6	136.0	150.0	167.7	184.4	198.7	210.4	209.2	212.8
Medicaid (Title XIX)	73.7	93.2	108.2	122.4	134.4	144.9	152.2	160.8	169.0	183.5
CHIP (Title XIX and Title XXI)	0.0	0.0	0.0	0.0	0.0	0.0	0.0	0.0	0.4	1.7
Department of Defense	10.4	11.5	11.6	12.0	11.8	12.0	12.0	12.1	12.2	12.7
Department of Veterans Affairs	10.9	11.9	12.6	13.6	14.6	14.8	15.6	15.5	16.3	17.5
Other third party payers and programs	**77.4**	**82.7**	**88.3**	**93.8**	**97.5**	**101.1**	**105.1**	**110.3**	**117.1**	**121.4**
Worksite healthcare	2.2	2.3	2.5	2.6	2.7	2.8	2.9	3.1	3.2	3.3
Other private revenues[2]	29.5	31.9	34.3	36.8	38.7	42.8	46.4	51.0	56.1	58.2
Indian health services	1.0	1.2	1.4	1.5	1.5	1.7	1.6	1.7	1.8	1.8
Workers' compensation	17.5	19.0	21.1	22.6	22.2	21.9	22.1	22.1	22.4	23.9
General assistance	5.0	5.2	5.5	5.0	5.5	5.4	5.4	5.2	4.9	3.9
Maternal/Child health	1.6	1.8	2.0	2.1	2.2	2.2	2.2	2.4	2.4	2.5
Vocational rehabilitation	0.3	0.3	0.3	0.3	0.4	0.4	0.4	0.4	0.4	0.4
Other federal programs[3]	1.5	1.8	2.0	2.2	2.4	2.5	2.8	3.1	3.4	3.8

(continued)

Table 5.2a. *(continued)*

Source of Funds	1990	1991	1992	1993	1994	1995	1996	1997	1998	1999
Substance abuse and mental health services administration	1.4	1.7	1.7	1.7	1.9	2.1	1.8	1.5	2.0	2.4
Other state and local programs[4]	15.9	16.2	16.1	17.4	18.5	17.6	17.5	17.8	18.4	18.8
School health	1.3	1.4	1.4	1.6	1.7	1.8	1.9	2.0	2.2	2.3
Public health activity[5]	20.0	22.1	24.4	26.8	29.6	31.0	32.4	34.8	37.5	40.7
Investment	48.7	52.0	56.9	61.2	63.9	65.9	67.7	72.2	80.1	86.8
Research[6]	12.7	13.8	15.1	16.5	17.8	18.7	17.8	19.6	21.5	23.4
Structures & equipment[7]	36.0	38.2	41.8	44.7	46.2	47.2	49.9	52.5	58.6	63.5

[1] Average annual growth from prior year shown.

[2] The most common source of other private funds is philanthropy. Philanthropic support may be direct from individuals or may be obtained through philanthropic fund-raising organizations such as the United Way. Support may also be obtained from foundations or corporations.

[3] Includes general hospital/medical, general hospital/medical NEC, non-XIX federal, and O.E.O.

[4] Includes non-XIX state and local, temporary disability insurance, and state and local subsidies.

[5] Governments are involved in organizing and delivering publicly provided health services such as epidemiological surveillance, inoculations, immunization/vaccination services, disease prevention programs, the operation of public health laboratories, and other such functions. In the NHEA, spending for these activities is reported in government public health activity.

[6] Research shown in the NHEA is that of non-profit or government entities. Research and development expenditures by drug and medical supply and equipment manufacturers are not shown in this line, as those expenditures are treated as intermediate purchases under the definitions of national income accounting; that is, the value of that research is deemed to be recouped through product sales.

[7] The structures component of the NHEA is defined as the value of new construction put in place by the medical sector. This measure of the medical sector includes establishments engaged in providing healthcare, but does not include retail establishments that sell non-durable or durable medical goods. The construction measure includes new buildings; additions, alterations, and major replacements; mechanical and electric installations; and site preparation.

Source: U.S. Centers for Medicare and Medicaid Services, Office of the Actuary, "National Health Expenditure Group."

For more information:

http://www.cms.gov/NationalHealthExpendData/

Internet release date: 09/30/2011

Table 5.2b. National Health Expenditures by Source of Funds: 2000 to 2009

(In billions of dollars [724.0 represents $724,000,000,000], except percent. Excludes Puerto Rico and Island Areas.)

Source of Funds	2000	2001	2002	2003	2004	2005	2006	2007	2008	2009
National health expenditure, total	**1,378.0**	**1,495.3**	**1,637.0**	**1,772.2**	**1,894.7**	**2,021.0**	**2,152.1**	**2,283.5**	**2,391.4**	**2,486.3**
Annual percent change[1]	7.1	8.5	9.5	8.3	6.9	6.7	6.5	6.1	4.7	4.0
Percent of gross domestic product	13.8	14.5	15.4	15.9	16.0	16.0	16.1	16.2	16.6	17.6
Out-of-pocket	202.1	209.5	222.8	237.1	248.8	263.8	272.1	289.4	298.2	299.3
Health insurance	918.8	1,013.5	1,119.5	1,219.2	1,316.2	1,410.5	1,513.7	1,597.5	1,681.8	1,767.4
Private health insurance	458.2	501.1	559.4	612.3	653.7	697.2	733.6	763.8	790.6	801.2
Medicare	224.4	247.4	264.8	282.4	311.3	339.9	403.1	431.4	465.7	502.3
Medicaid (Title XIX)	200.5	224.3	248.2	269.4	291.2	309.5	307.1	327.0	343.1	373.9
CHIP (Title XIX and Title XXI)	3.0	4.2	5.5	6.3	7.1	7.5	8.3	9.1	10.2	11.1
Department of Defense	13.7	15.4	18.9	22.3	24.9	26.5	29.7	32.2	33.9	36.5
Department of Veterans Affairs	19.1	21.1	22.8	26.5	28.0	29.8	31.9	34.0	38.2	42.4
Other third party payers and programs	124.5	130.9	137.3	148.2	153.9	159.8	168.5	179.5	181.2	186.1
Worksite healthcare	3.5	3.6	3.7	3.9	4.0	4.2	4.3	4.4	4.4	4.4
Other private revenues[2]	57.5	56.4	58.5	63.7	65.7	69.7	76.9	85.5	81.3	83.8
Indian health services	2.0	2.2	2.2	2.3	2.5	2.5	2.6	2.7	2.8	3.2
Workers' compensation	26.2	29.7	31.5	33.9	34.7	34.9	34.9	35.4	38.9	39.6
General assistance	3.9	4.8	5.1	5.6	5.9	6.2	6.7	6.9	7.1	7.1
Maternal/Child health	2.7	2.7	2.7	2.7	2.6	2.6	2.7	2.8	2.9	3.0
Vocational rehabilitation	0.4	0.4	0.5	0.5	0.5	0.5	0.5	0.5	0.5	0.5
Other federal programs[3]	4.5	5.3	5.7	6.0	6.2	6.3	6.4	6.7	6.9	7.3

(continued)

Table 5.2b. (continued)

Source of Funds	2000	2001	2002	2003	2004	2005	2006	2007	2008	2009
Substance abuse and mental health services administration	2.6	2.8	3.0	3.1	3.2	3.1	3.2	3.3	3.2	3.2
Other state and local programs[4]	18.7	20.3	21.6	23.6	25.4	26.4	26.8	27.4	28.9	29.4
School health	2.5	2.7	2.9	3.0	3.2	3.4	3.6	3.9	4.2	4.5
Public health activity[5]	43.0	47.5	51.9	53.7	54.0	56.2	62.6	68.8	72.9	77.2
Investment	89.6	94.0	105.4	114.0	121.8	130.7	135.2	148.4	157.2	156.2
Research[6]	25.5	28.5	32.0	34.9	38.5	40.3	41.4	41.9	43.2	45.3
Structures & equipment[7]	64.1	65.5	73.4	79.2	83.3	90.4	93.8	106.4	114.0	110.9

[1] Average annual growth from prior year shown.

[2] The most common source of other private funds is philanthropy. Philanthropic support may be direct from individuals or may be obtained through philanthropic fund-raising organizations such as the United Way. Support may also be obtained from foundations or corporations.

[3] Includes general hospital/medical, general hospital/medical NEC, non-XIX federal, and O.E.O.

[4] Includes non-XIX state and local, temporary disability insurance, and state and local subsidies.

[5] Governments are involved in organizing and delivering publicly provided health services such as epidemiological surveillance, inoculations, immunization/vaccination services, disease prevention programs, the operation of public health laboratories, and other such functions. In the NHEA, spending for these activities is reported in government public health activity.

[6] Research shown in the NHEA is that of non-profit or government entities. Research and development expenditures by drug and medical supply and equipment manufacturers are not shown in this line, as those expenditures are treated as intermediate purchases under the definitions of national income accounting; that is, the value of that research is deemed to be recouped through product sales.

[7] The structures component of the NHEA is defined as the value of new construction put in place by the medical sector. This measure of the medical sector includes establishments engaged in providing healthcare, but does not include retail establishments that sell non-durable or durable medical goods. The construction measure includes new buildings; additions, alterations, and major replacements; mechanical and electric installations; and site preparation.

Source: U. S. Centers for Medicare and Medicaid Services, Office of the Actuary, "National Health Expenditure Group."

For more information:

http://www.cms.gov/NationalHealthExpendData/

Internet release date: 09/30/2011

Table 5.3a. Hospital Care, Physician and Clinical Services, Nursing Care Facilities and Continuing Care Retirement Communities, and Prescription Drug Expenditures by Source of Funds: 1990 to 1999

(In billions of dollars [250.4 represents $250,400,000,000]. Excludes Puerto Rico and Island Areas.)

Source of funds	1990	1991	1992	1993	1994	1995	1996	1997	1998	1999
Hospital care, total	250.4	275.8	298.5	315.7	328.4	339.3	350.8	363.4	374.9	393.6
Out-of-pocket	11.2	11.9	12.3	12.1	10.7	10.1	10.2	10.9	11.9	12.7
Health insurance	206.8	229.7	251.1	267.6	280.5	292.5	303.4	313.1	320.9	337.8
Private health insurance	96.5	102.1	105.6	107.0	107.0	107.1	108.4	112.4	119.5	128.3
Medicare	67.8	73.8	83.7	92.2	100.6	109.1	116.6	122.0	120.1	122.2
Medicaid	26.7	36.5	43.9	49.5	53.7	56.8	58.9	59.6	61.8	66.9
Other health insurance[1]	15.8	17.3	17.8	18.9	19.3	19.5	19.5	19.1	19.5	20.4
Other third party payers and programs[2]	32.4	34.2	35.1	36.1	37.2	36.7	37.3	39.4	42.1	43.2
Physician and clinical services, total	158.9	176.5	191.3	202.8	212.2	222.3	231.3	242.9	257.9	271.1
Out-of-pocket	30.2	30.8	30.4	29.4	27.8	26.2	27.0	28.6	30.1	30.9
Health insurance	107.5	122.4	135.2	146.4	156.8	167.1	174.3	182.7	193.6	204.5
Private health insurance	67.2	78.1	87.3	95.2	101.1	106.8	111.0	115.6	123.0	128.4
Medicare	30.0	31.5	33.1	34.7	38.1	41.4	43.7	46.3	49.1	52.9
Medicaid	7.0	9.1	11.2	12.7	13.7	14.8	15.2	16.3	16.7	17.5
Other health insurance[1]	3.3	3.7	3.7	3.8	3.9	4.1	4.4	4.5	4.7	5.7
Other third party payers and programs[2]	21.2	23.3	25.6	26.9	27.6	29.0	30.0	31.6	34.3	35.8
Nursing care facilities and continuing care retirement communities, total	44.9	49.4	53.1	56.0	58.6	64.5	69.6	74.4	79.4	80.8

(continued)

217

Table 5.3a. (continued)

Source of funds	1990	1991	1992	1993	1994	1995	1996	1997	1998	1999
Out-of-pocket	18.1	18.4	18.6	18.5	17.8	19.7	20.1	21.6	25.8	26.4
Health insurance	21.9	25.6	28.7	31.4	35.2	38.2	42.6	45.4	47.0	47.7
Private health insurance	2.8	3.0	3.1	3.2	4.1	5.5	6.6	7.0	7.6	7.9
Medicare	1.7	2.0	2.9	4.0	5.6	6.7	8.4	10.0	10.4	9.0
Medicaid	16.4	19.6	21.5	22.8	24.0	24.5	26.0	26.8	27.3	29.1
Other health insurance[1]	1.0	1.1	1.2	1.3	1.5	1.5	1.6	1.6	1.7	1.8
Other third party payers and programs[2]	4.9	5.3	5.8	6.2	5.6	6.5	6.9	7.3	6.6	6.6
Prescription drugs, total	40.3	44.4	47.0	49.6	53.1	59.8	68.1	77.6	88.4	104.7
Out-of-pocket	22.9	23.6	23.7	23.9	23.3	23.3	24.5	26.0	27.8	30.9
Health insurance	16.2	19.6	22.1	24.5	28.5	35.1	42.3	50.1	58.9	71.9
Private health insurance	10.9	13.2	14.8	16.2	19.1	24.4	29.9	35.9	42.3	51.9
Medicare	0.2	0.2	0.3	0.4	0.5	0.7	1.0	1.3	1.6	1.9
Medicaid	5.1	6.0	6.9	7.7	8.6	9.7	10.8	12.2	14.0	16.6
Other health insurance[1]	0.1	0.1	0.1	0.2	0.2	0.3	0.5	0.7	1.0	1.5
Other third party payers and programs[2]	1.2	1.2	1.3	1.2	1.3	1.4	1.4	1.5	1.7	1.9

[1]Includes Children's Health Insurance Program (Titles XIX and XXI), Department of Defense, and Department of Veterans Affairs.
[2]Includes worksite healthcare, other private revenues, Indian Health Service, workers' compensation, general assistance, maternal and child health, vocational rehabilitation, other federal programs, Substance Abuse and Mental Health Services Administration, other state and local programs, and school health.
Source: U.S. Centers for Medicare and Medicaid Services, Office of the Actuary, "National Health Statistics Group."
For more information:
http://www.cms.gov/NationalHealthExpendData/
Internet release date: 09/30/2011

218

Table 5.3b. Hospital Care, Physician and Clinical Services, Nursing Care Facilities and Continuing Care Retirement Communities, and Prescription Drug Expenditures by Source of Funds: 2000 to 2009

(In billions of dollars [250.4 represents $250,400,000,000]. Excludes Puerto Rico and Island Areas.)

Source of funds	2000	2001	2002	2003	2004	2005	2006	2007	2008	2009
Hospital care, total	415.5	449.4	486.5	525.8	564.5	606.5	648.3	686.8	722.1	759.1
Out-of-pocket	13.4	13.7	15.0	16.4	17.6	19.0	20.3	21.6	23.2	24.4
Health insurance	358.3	390.9	425.3	458.4	493.8	532.1	567.2	598.8	634.0	669.3
Private health insurance	140.8	153.0	169.1	185.0	198.9	214.5	234.0	245.1	258.8	265.9
Medicare	124.4	136.4	145.3	152.9	165.3	179.1	187.1	195.3	208.1	220.4
Medicaid	71.2	77.7	84.9	90.7	97.7	104.8	110.2	119.7	123.6	136.1
Other health insurance[1]	21.9	23.8	26.0	29.8	32.0	33.7	36.0	38.8	43.6	47.0
Other third party payers and programs[2]	43.8	44.7	46.2	51.0	53.1	55.4	60.8	66.3	64.9	65.3
Physician and clinical services, total	290.0	314.7	340.8	368.4	393.6	419.6	441.6	462.6	486.5	505.9
Out-of-pocket	32.4	33.8	35.6	37.7	39.9	43.2	45.1	47.1	48.4	47.9
Health insurance	221.7	242.5	265.0	287.7	309.9	331.7	350.3	367.1	389.0	407.3
Private health insurance	137.8	150.2	164.5	178.7	190.2	204.8	214.2	223.2	233.3	237.7
Medicare	57.9	62.9	66.8	72.7	79.8	84.7	90.0	94.2	102.0	109.4
Medicaid	19.2	21.4	23.9	25.2	27.7	29.8	31.6	33.2	35.7	39.9
Other health insurance[1]	6.8	8.0	9.7	11.1	12.1	12.4	14.5	16.4	18.1	20.3
Other third party payers and programs[2]	35.9	38.4	40.3	43.0	43.9	44.7	46.2	48.4	49.0	50.6
Nursing care facilities and continuing care retirement communities, total	85.1	90.8	94.5	100.1	105.4	112.1	117.0	126.5	132.8	137.0

(continued)

Table 5.3b. (continued)

Source of funds	2000	2001	2002	2003	2004	2005	2006	2007	2008	2009
Out-of-pocket	27.7	28.3	28.7	31.2	32.5	34.2	35.1	38.5	40.4	39.8
Health insurance	51.5	56.9	60.0	62.6	66.3	70.5	73.9	78.0	83.2	87.5
Private health insurance	7.6	7.9	8.4	7.7	7.0	7.5	8.7	9.2	10.0	10.5
Medicare	10.1	12.4	13.9	14.7	16.9	19.0	21.0	23.4	26.0	28.0
Medicaid	31.9	34.5	35.5	37.8	39.8	41.2	41.3	42.1	43.6	45.0
Other health insurance[1]	1.9	2.1	2.2	2.5	2.7	2.8	2.8	3.3	3.7	4.0
Other third party payers and programs[2]	6.0	5.6	5.8	6.3	6.6	7.4	8.0	10.0	9.2	9.7
Prescription drugs, total	**120.9**	**138.7**	**158.2**	**175.2**	**190.3**	**201.7**	**219.8**	**230.2**	**237.2**	**249.9**
Out-of-pocket	34.0	36.7	41.2	45.3	47.7	50.6	49.9	52.5	51.8	53.0
Health insurance	84.6	99.3	113.9	126.3	138.9	147.2	165.8	173.9	181.7	193.3
Private health insurance	60.7	70.6	79.6	85.7	93.1	99.6	99.2	101.5	103.3	108.6
Medicare	2.1	2.4	2.5	2.5	3.4	3.9	39.6	45.8	50.4	54.8
Medicaid	19.8	23.3	27.4	32.1	35.7	36.3	18.9	18.1	18.9	20.0
Other health insurance[1]	2.1	2.9	4.3	6.0	6.7	7.4	8.1	8.5	9.1	10.0
Other third party payers and programs[2]	2.3	2.7	3.1	3.6	3.7	3.9	4.1	3.8	3.7	3.6

[1]Includes Children's Health Insurance Program (Titles XIX and XXI), Department of Defense, and Department of Veterans Affairs.
[2]Includes worksite healthcare, other private revenues, Indian Health Service, workers' compensation, general assistance, maternal and child health, vocational rehabilitation, other federal programs, Substance Abuse and Mental Health Services Administration, other state and local programs, and school health.
Source: U.S. Centers for Medicare and Medicaid Services, Office of the Actuary, "National Health Statistics Group."
For more information:
http://www.cms.gov/NationalHealthExpendData/
Internet release date: 09/30/2011

Table 5.4. Average Annual Expenditures Per Consumer Unit for Healthcare
(In dollars, except percent.)

| | Healthcare, total | | | | | | | | Percent distribution | | |
Item	Amount	Percent of total expenditures	Average Annual Expenditures	Health insurance	Medical services	Drugs	Medical supplies	Drugs and medical supplies[1]	Health insurance	Medical services	Drugs and medical supplies[1]
2004	2,574	5.9	43,395	1,332	648	480	114	594	51.7	25.2	23.1
2005	2,664	5.7	46,409	1,361	677	521	105	626	51.1	25.4	23.5
2006	2,766	5.7	48,398	1,465	670	514	117	631	53.0	24.2	22.8
2007	2,853	5.7	49,638	1,545	709	481	118	599	54.2	24.9	21.0
2008	2,976	5.9	50,486	1,653	727	482	114	596	55.5	24.4	20.0
2009	3,126	6.4	49,067	1,785	736	486	119	605	57.1	23.5	19.4
Age of reference person:											
Under 25 years old	676	2.4	28,119	381	167	97	30	127	56.4	24.7	18.8
25 to 34 years old	1,805	3.9	46,494	1,083	466	195	61	256	60.0	25.8	14.2
35 to 44 years old	2,520	4.4	57,301	1,436	650	335	100	435	57.0	25.8	17.3
45 to 54 years old	3,173	5.4	58,708	1,688	862	485	139	624	53.2	27.2	19.7
55 to 64 years old	3,895	7.4	52,463	2,017	1,054	679	144	823	51.8	27.1	21.1
65 to 74 years old	4,906	11.4	42,957	3,042	818	865	181	1,046	62.0	16.7	21.3
75 years old and over	4,779	15.1	31,676	3,011	824	787	158	945	63.0	17.2	19.8

(continued)

Table 5.4. (continued)

Item	Healthcare, total								Percent distribution		
	Amount	Percent of total expenditures	Average Annual Expenditures	Health insurance	Medical services	Drugs	Medical supplies	Drugs and medical supplies[1]	Health insurance	Medical services	Drugs and medical supplies[1]
Race of reference person:											
White and other	3,314	6.5	50,957	1,875	797	515	127	642	56.6	24.0	19.4
Black	1,763	5.0	35,311	1,133	294	279	57	336	64.3	16.7	19.1
Origin of reference person:											
Hispanic	1,568	3.7	41,981	848	418	241	61	302	54.1	26.7	19.3
Non-Hispanic	3,335	6.7	50,015	1,910	779	519	126	645	57.3	23.4	19.3
Region of residence:											
Northeast	3,132	5.8	53,868	1,916	625	481	111	592	61.2	20.0	18.9
Midwest	3,272	7.0	46,551	1,845	780	508	139	647	56.4	23.8	19.8
South	3,030	6.6	45,749	1,730	672	521	108	629	57.1	22.2	20.8
West	3,128	5.9	53,005	1,703	889	414	122	536	54.4	28.4	17.1
Size of consumer unit:											
One person	2,007	6.8	29,405	1,169	446	326	67	393	58.2	22.2	19.6
Two or more persons	3,578	6.3	57,002	2,034	854	551	140	691	56.8	23.9	19.3
Two persons	4,021	7.8	51,650	2,332	855	673	161	834	58.0	21.3	20.7

Three persons	3,273	5.8	56,645	1,890	783	466	134	600	57.7	23.9	18.3
Four persons	3,300	5.0	65,503	1,772	981	441	105	546	53.7	29.7	16.5
Five persons or more	2,960	4.7	63,439	1,628	781	425	126	551	55.0	26.4	18.6
Income before taxes:										
Quintiles of income:										
Lowest 20 percent	1,628	7.5	21,611	978	323	274	53	327	60.1	3.3	20.1
Second 20 percent	2,491	7.9	31,382	1,524	437	448	82	530	61.2	3.3	21.3
Third 20 percent	3,069	7.5	41,150	1,825	642	503	99	602	59.5	3.2	19.6
Fourth 20 percent	3,762	6.6	56,879	2,080	995	536	151	687	55.3	4.0	18.3
Highest 20 percent	4,677	5.0	94,244	2,516	1,283	669	208	877	53.8	4.4	18.8
Education:										
Less than high school graduate	2,010	6.6	30,323	1,215	364	356	76	432	60.4	18.1	21.5
High school graduate	2,913	7.5	38,693	1,712	624	487	90	577	58.8	21.4	19.8
High school graduate with some college	2,917	6.5	44,697	1,635	691	487	105	592	56.1	23.7	20.3

(continued)

Table 5.4. (*continued*)

Item	Healthcare, total								Percent distribution		
	Amount	Percent of total expenditures	Average Annual Expenditures	Health insurance	Medical services	Drugs	Medical supplies	Drugs and medical supplies[1]	Health insurance	Medical services	Drugs and medical supplies[1]
Associate's degree	3,000	5.9	50,446	1,660	729	476	135	611	55.3	24.3	20.4
Bachelor's degree	3,778	5.7	65,908	2,121	974	525	157	682	56.1	25.8	18.1
Master's, professional, doctoral degree	4,503	5.9	76,072	2,544	1,177	591	191	782	56.5	26.1	17.4

[1]Includes prescription and nonprescription drugs.

Source: Bureau of Labor Statistics, Consumer Expenditure Survey, annual.
For more information:
http://www.bls.gov/cex/
http://www.bls.gov/cex/#tables/
Internet release date: 09/30/2011

Source: http://www.census.gov/compendia/statab/2012/tables/12s0143.pdf.

but is not as consistent a pattern for medical services. For that category, people between the ages of 55 and 64 have higher expenditures than those ages 65 to 74 and 75 and over.

Table 5.5 provides figures on health insurance coverage status for 2009 by such characteristics as age, sex, race, Hispanic origin, and household income. Actual numbers are provided along with percentages, and figures are presented for coverage by private or government health insurance, including Medicare and Medicaid. Looking at the income breakdowns, for example, the percentage covered by any insurance increases as income increases. This is because as income increases, the percentage of private health insurance increases from 27.2 percent for those earning less than $25,000 to 85 percent for those earning $75,000 or more. In contrast, the highest percentage of people with Medicaid coverage are those in the lowest income category.

Table 5.6 also includes information on persons with and without health insurance coverage but provides this information for just one year, 2009. Rather than examining these figures by individual characteristics, this table focuses on variation by state and also provides information about all persons not covered and also specifically whether children are covered.

Table 5.7 presents data showing the dramatic growth of the national healthcare expenditure segment of the United States economy from 1960 to 2011. It presents these figures broken down by personal healthcare, administration, net cost of private health insurance, public health, and investment costs of research, structures and equipment. Of particular importance in the health reform debate is growth in the percentage of the nation's GDP represented by the health sector from 5.2 percent in 1960 to 27.9 percent in 2011. Also relevant is the growth in the percentage of health expenditures spent on administration and net cost of private health insurance, which grew from 3.9 percent in 1960 to 7.0 percent in 2011.

Table 5.8 provides information on life expectancy at birth, as well as at ages 65 and 75. Data on life expectancy at birth is presented back to 1900, at 65 years back to 1950, and at age 75

Table 5.5. Health Insurance Coverage Status by Selected Characteristics: 2008 and 2009

Characteristic	Total persons	Number (1,000)							Percent				
		Total[1]	Covered by private or government health insurance					Not covered by health insurance	Total[1]	Covered by private or government health insurance			Not covered by health insurance
			Private		Government					Private	Medicaid	
			Total	Group health[2]	Medicare	Medicaid						
2008	301,483	255,143	200,992	176,332	43,029	42,641	46,340	84.6	66.7	14.1	15.4
2009	304,280	253,606	194,545	169,689	43,440	47,758	50,674	83.3	63.9	15.7	16.7
Age:												
Under 18 years	75,040	67,527	45,288	41,892	543	25,331	7,513	90.0	60.4	33.8	10.0
..Under 6 years	25,542	23,192	14,137	13,282	194	10,090	2,350	90.8	55.3	39.5	9.2
..6 to 11 years	24,613	22,268	15,077	14,167	193	8,294	2,344	90.5	61.3	33.7	9.5
..12 to 17 years	24,885	22,066	16,074	14,442	157	6,946	2,819	88.7	64.6	27.9	11.3
18 to 24 years	29,313	20,389	16,308	12,802	199	4,437	8,923	69.6	55.6	15.1	30.4
25 to 34 years	41,085	29,122	24,708	22,612	547	4,236	11,963	70.9	60.1	10.3	29.1
35 to 44 years	40,447	31,689	27,962	26,125	934	3,562	8,759	78.3	69.1	8.8	21.7
45 to 54 years	44,387	36,481	32,147	29,867	1,796	3,552	7,906	82.2	72.4	8.0	17.8
55 to 64 years	35,395	30,462	25,718	23,245	3,318	2,991	4,933	86.1	72.7	8.5	13.9

226

65 years and over	38,613	37,937	22,414	13,146	36,102	3,649	676	98.2	58.0	9.5	1.8

Sex:

Male	149,485	122,022	95,046	83,774	19,088	21,824	27,463	81.6	63.6	14.6	18.4
Female	154,795	131,584	99,498	85,915	24,352	25,934	23,211	85.0	64.3	16.8	15.0

Race:

White alone[3]	242,403	204,004	161,513	139,809	36,807	32,814	38,399	84.2	66.6	13.5	15.8
Black alone[3]	38,624	30,522	18,813	17,275	4,598	10,459	8,102	79.0	48.7	27.1	21.0
Asian alone[3]	14,011	11,602	9,352	8,180	1,304	1,951	2,409	82.8	66.7	13.9	17.2
Hispanic origin[4]	48,901	33,081	19,453	17,830	3,274	12,959	15,820	67.6	39.8	26.5	32.4

Household income:

Less than $25,000	58,159	42,675	15,795	9,350	14,986	21,693	15,483	73.4	27.2	37.3	26.6
$25,000–$49,999	71,340	56,062	38,211	31,199	13,821	14,363	15,278	78.6	53.6	20.1	21.4
$50,000–$74,999	58,381	49,029	41,689	37,376	6,640	6,066	9,352	84.0	71.4	10.4	16.0
$75,000 or more	116,400	105,839	98,849	91,765	7,993	5,636	10,561	90.9	84.9	4.8	9.1
Persons below poverty	43,569	29,666	8,599	5,437	4,996	19,919	13,903	68.1	19.7	45.7	31.9

(continued)

(continued)

[1]Includes other government insurance not shown separately. Persons with coverage counted only once in total, even though they may have been covered by more than that one type of policy.

[2]Related to employment of self or other family members.

[3]Refers to people who reported specified race and did not report any other race category.

[4]Persons of Hispanic origin may be of any race.

Source: U.S. Census Bureau, Income, Poverty, and Health Insurance Coverage in the United States: 2009, Current Population Reports, P60-238, September 2010; Table HI01, "Health Insurance Data, Health Insurance Coverage Status and Type of Coverage by Selected Characteristics: 2009" and Table HI03, "Health Insurance Coverage Status and Type of Coverage by Selected Characteristics for Poor People in the Poverty Universe: 2009."

For more information:

http://www.census.gov/hhes/www/hlthins/hlthins.html

http://www.census.gov/hhes/www/cpstables/032010/health/toc.htm

Internet release date: 09/30/2011

Source: http://www.census.gov/compendia/statab/2012/tables/12s0155.pdf.

Table 5.6. Persons with and without Health Insurance Coverage by State, 2009

(253,606 represents 253,606,000. Based on the Current Population Survey, Annual Social and Economic Supplement [CPS ASES]; see text, Section 1, Population, and Appendix III)

State	Total Persons covered (1,000)	Total persons not covered		Children not covered	
		Number (1,000)	Percent of total	Number (1,000)	Percent of total
United States	253,606	50,674	16.7	7,513	10.0
Alabama	3,880	789	16.9	86	7.9
Alaska	568	122	17.7	19	9.9
Arizona	5,239	1,273	19.6	229	13.4
Arkansas	2,304	548	19.2	81	11.5
California	29,449	7,345	20.0	1,012	10.7
Colorado	4,209	762	15.3	119	9.6
Connecticut	3,062	418	12.0	62	7.7
Delaware	766	118	13.4	19	8.8
District of Columbia	522	74	12.4	9	8.0
Florida	14,287	4,118	22.4	724	17.9
Georgia	7,687	1,985	20.5	293	11.3
Hawaii	1,149	102	8.2	11	3.5
Idaho	1,294	232	15.2	43	10.2
Illinois	10,875	1,891	14.8	291	9.1
Indiana	5,462	902	14.2	141	8.6
Iowa	2,654	342	11.4	42	5.9
Kansas	2,380	365	13.3	58	8.1
Kentucky	3,588	694	16.2	84	8.2
Louisiana	3,741	711	16.0	97	8.4
Maine	1,167	133	10.2	11	4.0
Maryland	4,874	793	14.0	94	7.0
Massachusetts	6,337	295	4.4	43	2.9
Michigan	8,465	1,350	13.8	132	5.6
Minnesota	4,747	456	8.8	68	5.5
Mississippi	2,349	502	17.6	85	10.9
Missouri	5,055	914	15.3	139	9.7
Montana	823	149	15.4	23	10.4
Nebraska	1,574	205	11.5	31	6.7
Nevada	2,086	546	20.8	89	13.3
	1,176	138	10.5	11	3.8

(continued)

229

Table 5.6.   (*continued*)

State	Total Persons covered (1,000)	Total persons not covered		Children not covered	
		Number (1,000)	Percent of total	Number (1,000)	Percent of total
New Hampshire					
New Jersey	7,309	1,371	15.8	190	9.2
New Mexico	1,548	430	21.7	72	14.0
New York	16,347	2,837	14.8	335	7.5
North Carolina	7,663	1,685	18.0	276	11.8
North Dakota	565	67	10.7	9	5.9
Ohio	9,819	1,643	14.3	237	8.7
Oklahoma	2,977	659	18.1	117	12.6
Oregon	3,156	678	17.7	103	11.9
Pennsylvania	11,004	1,409	11.4	193	6.8
Rhode Island	906	127	12.3	14	6.0
South Carolina	3,740	766	17.0	136	12.3
South Dakota	693	108	13.5	17	8.4
Tennessee	5,290	963	15.4	98	6.6
Texas	18,224	6,433	26.1	1,150	16.5
Utah	2,385	415	14.8	99	11.3
Vermont	557	61	9.9	7	5.6
Virginia	6,764	1,014	13.0	144	7.5
Washington	5,845	869	12.9	75	4.8
West Virginia	1,552	253	14.0	24	6.2
Wisconsin	5,037	527	9.5	61	4.7
Wyoming	455	86	15.8	13	9.6

Source: U.S. Census Bureau, Income, Poverty, and Health Insurance Coverage in the United States: 2009, Current Population Reports, P60-238, 2010, Table HI05, "Health Insurance Coverage Status and Type of Coverage by State and age for all People: 2009."
For more information:
http://www.census.gov/hhes/www/hlthins.html
http://www.census.gov/hhes/www/cpstables/032010/health/toc.htm
Internet release date: 09\30\2011
Source: http://www.census.gov/compendia/statab/2012/tables/12s0155.pdf.

back to 1980. The information is presented by sex and for whites, blacks, and Hispanics. Several important trends are shown that significantly affect the healthcare system and its reform. The increase in the expectation of life remaining at the

Table 5.7. Gross Domestic Product, National Health Expenditures, Per Capita Amounts, Percent Distribution, and Average Annual Percent Change: United States, Selected Years, 1960–2011

(Data are compiled from various sources by the Centers for Medicare & Medicaid Services)

Gross domestic product and national health expenditures	1960	1970	1980	1990	2000	2005	2010	2011
			Amount, in billions					
Gross domestic product (GDP)	$526	$1,038	$2,788	$5,801	$9,952	$12,623	$14,499	$15,076
			Deflator (2005 = 100.0)					
Price deflator for GDP[1]	18.6	24.3	47.8	72.3	88.7	100.0	111.0	113.4
			Amount, in billions					
National health expenditures..........	$27.4	$74.9	$255.8	$724.3	$1,377.2	$2,030.5	$2,600.0	$2,700.7
Health consumption expenditures	24.8	67.1	235.7	675.6	1,289.6	1,904.0	2,450.8	2,547.2
Personal healthcare	23.4	63.1	217.2	616.8	1,165.4	1,697.1	2,190.0	2,279.3
Administration and net cost of private health insurance...........................	1.1	2.6	12.0	38.8	81.2	150.9	181.5	188.9
Public health	0.4	1.4	6.4	20.0	43.0	56.0	79.3	79.0
Investment[2]	2.6	7.8	20.1	48.7	87.5	126.5	149.1	153.5
			Deflator (2005 = 100.0)					
Chain-weighted national health expenditure deflator[1]	—	—	—	—	—	100.0	114.6	117.3
			Per capita amount, in dollars					
National health expenditures............	$147	$356	$1,110	$2,854	$4,878	$6,875	$8,417	$8,680

(continued)

Table 5.7. (continued)

Gross domestic product and national health expenditures	1960	1970	1980	1990	2000	2005	2010	2011
Health consumption expenditures	133	319	1,023	2,662	4,568	6,447	7,934	8,187
Personal healthcare	125	300	943	2,430	4,128	5,746	7,090	7,326
Administration and net cost of private health insurance	6	12	52	153	288	511	588	607
Public health	2	6	28	79	152	190	257	254
Investment[2]	14	37	87	192	310	428	483	493
Percent								
National health expenditures as percent of GDP	5.2	7.2	9.2	12.5	13.8	16.1	17.9	17.9
Percent distribution								
National health expenditures	100.0	100.0	100.0	100.0	100.0	100.0	100.0	100.0
Health consumption expenditures	90.6	89.6	92.1	93.3	93.6	93.8	94.3	94.3
Personal healthcare	85.4	84.3	84.9	85.2	84.6	83.6	84.2	84.4
Administration and net cost of private health insurance	3.9	3.5	4.7	5.4	5.9	7.4	7.0	7.0
Public health	1.4	1.8	2.5	2.8	3.1	2.8	3.1	2.9
Investment[2]	9.4	10.4	7.9	6.7	6.4	6.2	5.7	5.7
Average annual percent change from previous year shown[3]								
GDP	...	7.0	10.4	7.6	5.5	4.9	2.8	4.0

National health expenditures............	...	10.6	13.1	11.0	6.6	8.1	5.1	3.9
Health consumption expenditures	...	10.5	13.4	11.1	6.7	8.1	5.2	3.9
Personal healthcare	...	10.4	13.2	11.0	6.6	7.8	5.2	4.1
Administration and net cost of private health insurance............	...	9.4	16.4	12.4	7.7	13.2	3.8	4.1
Public health	...	13.8	16.9	12.0	8.0	5.4	7.2	-0.5
Investment²	...	11.7	10.0	9.2	6.0	7.6	3.3	2.9
National health expenditures, per capita.......	...	9.3	12.0	9.9	5.5	7.1	4.1	3.1
Health consumption expenditures	...	9.1	12.4	10.0	5.5	7.1	4.2	3.2
Personal healthcare	...	9.1	12.1	9.9	5.4	6.8	4.3	3.3
Administration and net cost of private health insurance............	...	8.1	15.4	11.3	6.5	12.2	2.8	3.3
Public health	...	12.5	15.8	10.9	6.8	4.4	6.3	-1.2
Investment²	...	10.4	8.9	8.2	4.9	6.7	2.4	2.2

—Data not available.

—Category not applicable.

[1]Year 2005 = 100.

[2]Investment consists of research and structures and equipment.

[3]See Appendix II, Average annual rate of change (percent change).

NOTES: Dollar amounts shown are in current dollars.

Deflating healthcare spending separates the effects of price growth from growth attributable to all other factors. *(continued)*

(continued)

The dollar value of these estimates of real healthcare expenditures is determined by the index(es) chosen to remove price growth from spending.

One approach to deflating health spending is to remove the effects of economy-wide inflation alone using the GDP deflator.

An alternative approach to removing the effects of price growth from health spending for the National Health Expenditure Accounts is to deflate healthcare expenditures by a measure of medical specific price inflation.

For personal healthcare (PHC) spending, this would involve directly deflating expenditures by price indexes associated with the services and goods provided; for non-PHC spending this would involve deflating by composite indexes matching the components of spending for each category.

For more information on the detailed price series recommended for deflating each category of spending, see the National Health Expenditure Accounts Methodology Paper, 2011.

Available from:

http://www.cms.gov/Research-Statistics-Data-and-Systems/Statistics-Trends-and-Reports/NationalHealthExpendData/Downloads/dsm-11.pdf.

The data reflect preliminary annual estimates of the resident population of the United States as of July 1, 2011, excluding the Armed Forces overseas.

See Appendix II, Gross domestic product (GDP); Health expenditures, national.

Percents are calculated using unrounded data.

Estimates may not add to totals because of rounding.

Starting with Health, United States, 2010, estimates are based on a revised methodology that incorporates available source data and various methodological and definitional changes. These revisions are due to a comprehensive change in the classification structure of how estimates are defined and presented. For more information on the impact of these revisions, see: http://www.cms.gov/NationalHealthExpendData/downloads/benchmark2009.pdf.

Data have been revised and differ from previous editions of Health, United States.

SOURCE: Centers for Medicare & Medicaid Services, Office of the Actuary, National Health Statistics Group, National Health Expenditure Accounts, National health expenditures aggregate, 1960–2011. Available from: http://www.cms.gov/Research-Statistics-Data-and-Systems/Statistics-Trends-and-Reports/NationalHealthExpendData/index.html?redirect=/nationalhealthexpenddata/;

U.S. Department of Commerce Bureau of Economic Analysis, National Economic Accounts, National Income and Product Accounts, Table 1.1.9, accessed on May 16, 2013. Available from: http://www.bea.gov/iTable/iTable.cfm?ReqID=9&step=1

See Appendix I, National Health Expenditure Accounts (NHEA); National Income and Product Accounts (NIPA).

Health, United States, 2013

Source: http://www.cdc.gov/nchs/data/hus/2013/112.pdf.

Table 5.8. Life Expectancy at Birth, at Age 65, and at Age 75, by Sex, Race, and Hispanic Origin: United States, Selected Years, 1900–2010[1]

Specified age and year	All races			White			Black or African American[1]		
	Both sexes	Male	Female	Both sexes	Male	Female	Both sexes	Male	Female
At birth				Life expectancy, in years					
1900[2,3].........	47.3	46.3	48.3	47.6	46.6	48.7	33.0	32.5	33.5
1950[3]...........	68.2	65.6	71.1	69.1	66.5	72.2	60.8	59.1	62.9
1960[3]...........	69.7	66.6	73.1	70.6	67.4	74.1	63.6	61.1	66.3
1970.............	70.8	67.1	74.7	71.7	68.0	75.6	64.1	60.0	68.3
1975.............	72.6	68.8	76.6	73.4	69.5	77.3	66.8	62.4	71.3
1980.............	73.7	70.0	77.4	74.4	70.7	78.1	68.1	63.8	72.5
1981.............	74.1	70.4	77.8	74.8	71.1	78.4	68.9	64.5	73.2
1982.............	74.5	70.8	78.1	75.1	71.5	78.7	69.4	65.1	73.6
1983.............	74.6	71.0	78.1	75.2	71.6	78.7	69.4	65.2	73.5
1984.............	74.7	71.1	78.2	75.3	71.8	78.7	69.5	65.3	73.6
1985.............	74.7	71.1	78.2	75.3	71.8	78.7	69.3	65.0	73.4
1986.............	74.7	71.2	78.2	75.4	71.9	78.8	69.1	64.8	73.4
1987.............	74.9	71.4	78.3	75.6	72.1	78.9	69.1	64.7	73.4
1988.............	74.9	71.4	78.3	75.6	72.2	78.9	68.9	64.4	73.2
1989.............	75.1	71.7	78.5	75.9	72.5	79.2	68.8	64.3	73.3
1990.............	75.4	71.8	78.8	76.1	72.7	79.4	69.1	64.5	73.6

(continued)

235

Table 5.8. *(continued)*

Specified age and year	All races			White			Black or African American[1]		
	Both sexes	Male	Female	Both sexes	Male	Female	Both sexes	Male	Female
1991............	75.5	72.0	78.9	76.3	72.9	79.6	69.3	64.6	73.8
1992............	75.8	72.3	79.1	76.5	73.2	79.8	69.6	65.0	73.9
1993............	75.5	72.2	78.8	76.3	73.1	79.5	69.2	64.6	73.7
1994............	75.7	72.4	79.0	76.5	73.3	79.6	69.5	64.9	73.9
1995............	75.8	72.5	78.9	76.5	73.4	79.6	69.6	65.2	73.9
1996............	76.1	73.1	79.1	76.8	73.9	79.7	70.2	66.1	74.2
1997............	76.5	73.6	79.4	77.1	74.3	79.9	71.1	67.2	74.7
1998............	76.7	73.8	79.5	77.3	74.5	80.0	71.3	67.6	74.8
1999............	76.7	73.9	79.4	77.3	74.6	79.9	71.4	67.8	74.7
2000............	76.8	74.1	79.3	77.3	74.7	79.9	71.8	68.2	75.1
2001............	77.0	74.3	79.5	77.5	74.9	80.0	72.0	68.5	75.3
2002............	77.0	74.4	79.6	77.5	74.9	80.1	72.2	68.7	75.4
2003............	77.2	74.5	79.7	77.7	75.1	80.2	72.4	68.9	75.7
2004............	77.6	75.0	80.1	78.1	75.5	80.5	72.9	69.4	76.1
2005............	77.6	75.0	80.1	78.0	75.5	80.5	73.0	69.5	76.2
2006............	77.8	75.2	80.3	78.3	75.8	80.7	73.4	69.9	76.7
2007............	78.1	75.5	80.6	78.5	76.0	80.9	73.8	70.3	77.0
2008............	78.2	75.6	80.6	78.5	76.1	80.9	74.3	70.9	77.3
2009............	78.5	76.0	80.9	78.8	76.4	81.2	74.7	71.4	77.7

	78.7	76.2	81.0	78.9	76.5	81.3	75.1	71.8	78.0
2010.............									

At 65 years

1950³.........	13.9	12.8	15.0	14.1	12.8	15.1	13.9	12.9	14.9
1960³.........	14.3	12.8	15.8	14.4	12.9	15.9	13.9	12.7	15.1
1970..........	15.2	13.1	17.0	15.2	13.1	17.1	14.2	12.5	15.7
1975..........	16.1	13.8	18.1	16.1	13.8	18.2	15.0	13.1	16.7
1980..........	16.4	14.1	18.3	16.5	14.2	18.4	15.1	13.0	16.8
1981..........	16.6	14.3	18.6	16.7	14.4	18.7	15.5	13.4	17.2
1982..........	16.8	14.5	18.7	16.9	14.5	18.8	15.7	13.5	17.5
1983..........	16.7	14.4	18.6	16.8	14.5	18.7	15.4	13.2	17.2
1984..........	16.8	14.5	18.6	16.8	14.6	18.7	15.4	13.2	17.2
1985..........	16.7	14.5	18.5	16.8	14.5	18.7	15.2	13.0	16.9
1986..........	16.8	14.6	18.6	16.9	14.7	18.7	15.2	13.0	17.0
1987..........	16.9	14.7	18.7	17.0	14.8	18.8	15.2	13.0	17.0
1988..........	16.9	14.7	18.6	17.0	14.8	18.7	15.1	12.9	16.9
1989..........	17.1	15.0	18.8	17.2	15.1	18.9	15.2	13.0	16.9
1990..........	17.2	15.1	18.9	17.3	15.2	19.1	15.4	13.2	17.2
1991..........	17.4	15.3	19.1	17.5	15.4	19.2	15.5	13.4	17.2
1992..........	17.5	15.4	19.2	17.6	15.5	19.3	15.7	13.5	17.4
1993..........	17.3	15.3	18.9	17.4	15.4	19.0	15.5	13.4	17.1
1994..........	17.4	15.5	19.0	17.5	15.6	19.1	15.7	13.6	17.2
1995..........	17.4	15.6	18.9	17.6	15.7	19.1	15.6	13.6	17.1

(continued)

Table 5.8. (continued)

Specified age and year	All races			White			Black or African American[1]		
	Both sexes	Male	Female	Both sexes	Male	Female	Both sexes	Male	Female
1996	17.5	15.7	19.0	17.6	15.8	19.1	15.8	13.9	17.2
1997	17.7	15.9	19.2	17.8	16.0	19.3	16.1	14.2	17.6
1998	17.8	16.0	19.2	17.8	16.1	19.3	16.1	14.3	17.4
1999	17.7	16.1	19.1	17.8	16.1	19.2	16.0	14.3	17.3
2000	17.6	16.0	19.0	17.7	16.1	19.1	16.1	14.1	17.5
2001	17.9	16.2	19.2	18.0	16.3	19.3	16.2	14.2	17.7
2002	17.9	16.3	19.2	18.0	16.4	19.3	16.3	14.4	17.8
2003	18.1	16.5	19.3	18.2	16.6	19.4	16.5	14.5	18.0
2004	18.4	16.9	19.6	18.5	17.0	19.7	16.8	14.9	18.3
2005	18.4	16.9	19.6	18.5	17.0	19.7	16.9	15.0	18.3
2006	18.7	17.2	19.9	18.7	17.3	19.9	17.2	15.2	18.6
2007	18.8	17.4	20.0	18.9	17.4	20.1	17.3	15.4	18.8
2008	18.8	17.4	20.0	18.9	17.5	20.0	17.5	15.5	18.9
2009	19.1	17.7	20.3	19.2	17.7	20.3	17.8	15.9	19.2
2010	19.1	17.7	20.3	19.2	17.8	20.3	17.8	15.9	19.3
At 75 years									
1980	10.4	8.8	11.5	10.4	8.8	11.5	9.7	8.3	10.7
1981	10.6	9.0	11.7	10.6	9.0	11.7	10.4	9.0	11.4
1982	10.7	9.1	11.9	10.7	9.0	11.9	10.6	9.1	11.6

Year									
1983	10.6	9.0	11.7	10.6	8.9	11.7	10.3	8.9	11.4
1984	10.7	9.0	11.8	10.7	9.0	11.8	10.3	8.9	11.4
1985	10.6	9.0	11.7	10.6	9.0	11.7	10.1	8.7	11.1
1986	10.7	9.1	11.7	10.7	9.1	11.8	10.1	8.6	11.1
1987	10.7	9.1	11.8	10.7	9.1	11.8	10.1	8.6	11.1
1988	10.6	9.1	11.7	10.7	9.1	11.7	10.0	8.5	11.0
1989	10.9	9.3	11.9	10.9	9.3	11.9	10.1	8.6	11.0
1990	10.9	9.4	12.0	11.0	9.4	12.0	10.2	8.6	11.2
1991	11.1	9.5	12.1	11.1	9.5	12.1	10.2	8.7	11.2
1992	11.2	9.6	12.2	11.2	9.6	12.2	10.4	8.9	11.4
1993	10.9	9.5	11.9	11.0	9.5	12.0	10.2	8.7	11.1
1994	11.0	9.6	12.0	11.1	9.6	12.0	10.3	8.9	11.2
1995	11.0	9.7	11.9	11.1	9.7	12.0	10.2	8.8	11.1
1996	11.1	9.8	12.0	11.1	9.8	12.0	10.3	9.0	11.2
1997	11.2	9.9	12.1	11.2	9.9	12.1	10.7	9.3	11.5
1998	11.3	10.0	12.2	11.3	10.0	12.2	10.5	9.2	11.3
1999	11.2	10.0	12.1	11.2	10.0	12.1	10.4	9.2	11.1
2000	11.0	9.8	11.8	11.0	9.8	11.9	10.4	9.0	11.3
2001	11.2	9.9	12.0	11.2	10.0	12.1	10.5	9.0	11.5
2002	11.2	10.0	12.0	11.2	10.0	12.1	10.5	9.1	11.5
2003	11.3	10.1	12.1	11.3	10.2	12.1	10.7	8.7	11.6
2004	11.5	10.4	12.4	11.6	10.4	12.4	10.9	9.4	11.2

(continued)

Table 5.8. (continued)

Specified age and year	All races			White			Black or African American[1]		
	Both sexes	Male	Female	Both sexes	Male	Female	Both sexes	Male	Female
2005..............	11.5	10.4	12.3	11.5	10.4	12.3	10.9	9.4	11.2
2006..............	11.7	10.6	12.5	11.1	10.6	12.5	11.1	9.1	12.0
2007..............	11.9	10.7	12.6	11.9	10.8	12.6	11.2	9.8	12.1
2008..............	11.8	10.7	12.6	11.8	10.7	12.6	11.3	9.8	12.2
2009..............	12.1	11.0	12.9	12.1	10.4	12.9	11.6	10.2	12.5
2010..............	12.1	11.0	12.9	12.1	11.0	12.8	11.6	10.2	12.5

Specified age and year	White, not Hispanic			Black, not Hispanic			Hispanic[4]		
	Both sexes	Male	Female	Both sexes	Male	Female	Both sexes	Male	Female
	Life expectancy, in years								
At birth									
2006..............	78.2	75.7	80.6	73.1	69.5	76.4	80.3	77.5	82.9
2007..............	78.4	75.9	80.8	73.5	69.9	76.7	80.7	77.8	83.2
2008..............	78.4	76.0	80.7	73.9	70.5	77.0	80.8	78.0	83.3
2009..............	78.7	76.3	81.1	74.3	70.9	77.4	81.1	78.4	83.5
2010..............	78.8	76.4	81.1	74.7	71.4	77.7	81.2	78.5	83.8
At 65 years									
2006..............	18.7	17.2	19.9	17.1	15.1	18.5	20.2	18.5	21.5

2007.............	18.8	17.4	20.0	17.2	15.3	18.7	20.5	18.7	21.7
2008.............	18.8	17.4	20.0	17.4	15.4	18.8	20.4	18.7	21.6
2009.............	19.1	17.7	19.5	17.7	15.8	19.1	20.7	19.0	21.9
2010.............	19.1	17.7	20.3	17.7	15.8	19.1	20.6	18.8	22.0
At 75 years									
2006.............	11.7	10.6	12.5	11.1	9.6	12.0	13.0	11.7	13.7
2007.............	11.8	10.7	12.6	11.2	9.7	12.1	13.1	11.8	13.8
2008.............	11.8	10.7	12.6	11.3	9.8	12.2	13.0	11.7	13.8
2009.............	12.0	11.0	12.9	11.6	10.1	12.4	13.3	12.0	13.8
2010.............	12.0	11.0	12.8	11.6	10.1	12.5	13.2	11.7	14.1

[1]Data shown for 1900-1960 are for the nonwhite population.

[2]Death registration area only. The death registration area increased from 10 states and the District of Columbia (D.C.) in 1900 to the coterminous United States in 1933. See Appendix II, Registration area.

[3]Includes deaths of persons who were not residents of the 50 states and D.C.

[4]Hispanic origin was added to the U.S. standard death certificate in 1989 and was adopted by every state in 1997.

To estimate life expectancy, age-specific death rates were corrected to address racial and ethnic misclassification, which underestimates deaths in the Hispanic population.

Life expectancies for the Hispanic population are adjusted for underreporting on the death certificate of Hispanic ethnicity, but are not adjusted to account for the potential effects of return migration.

To address the effects of age misstatement at the oldest ages, the probability of death for Hispanic persons older than 80 years is estimated as a function of non-Hispanic white mortality with the use of the Brass relational logit model. See Appendix II, Hispanic origin.

See Appendix II, Race, for a discussion of sources of bias in death rates by race and Hispanic origin.

NOTES: Populations for computing life expectancy for 1991-1999 are 1990-based postcensal estimates of the U.S. resident population. Starting with Health, United States, 2012, populations for computing life expectancy for 2001-2009 were based on intercensal population estimates of the U.S. resident population.

Populations for computing life expectancy for 2010 were based on 2010 census counts. *(continued)*

(continued)

See Appendix I, Population Census and Population Estimates.

In 1997, life table methodology was revised to construct complete life tables by single years of age that extend to age 100. (Anderson RN. Method for constructing complete annual U.S. life tables. NCHS. Vital Health Stat 2(129). 1999.

Previously, abridged life tables were constructed for 5-year age groups ending with 85 years and over.

In 2000, the life table methodology was revised. The revised methodology is similar to that developed for the 1999-2001 decennial life tables. In 2008, the life table methodology was further refined.

See Appendix II, Life expectancy.

Starting with 2003 data, some states allowed the reporting of more than one race on the death certificate.

The multiple-race data for these states were bridged to the single-race categories of the 1977 Office of Management and Budget standards, for comparability with other states.

The race groups, white and black include persons of Hispanic and non-Hispanic origin. Persons of Hispanic origin may be of any race. See Appendix II, Race.

Data for additional years are available. See the Excel spreadsheet on the Health, United States website at: http://www.cdc.gov/nchs/hus.htm.

SOURCE: CDC/NCHS, National Vital Statistics System, public-use Mortality Files; Grove RD, Hetzel AM. Vital statistics rates in the United States, 1940-1960. Washington, DC: U.S. Government Printing Office, 1968; Arias E. United States life tables by Hispanic origin. Vital health statistics; vol 2 no 152. Hyattsville, MD: NCHS. 2010. Murphy SL, Xu JQ, Kochanek KD. Deaths: Final data for 2010. National vital statistics reports; vol 61 no 4. Hyattsville, MD: NCHS; 2012. Available from: http://www.cdc.gov/nchs/data/nvsr/nvsr61_04.pdf.

See Appendix I, National Vital Statistics System (NVSS).

Health, United States, 2013

Source: http://www.cdc.gov/nchs/data/hus/2013/018.pdf.

age 65 from 1959 to 1961 to 2018 of over four years for males and for five years for women greatly increases the cost of health-care in general and specifically of Medicare, the federal health insurance program for older adults. Also notable is the differ-ence in life expectancy between whites, blacks, and Hispanics. In general, the best life expectancies are for Hispanics, followed by whites and then blacks.

These tables are examples of the vast wealth of data provided by the federal government. These tables were selected both to provide an example of the type of data available and because together, they provide a good starting point in the use of data to understand the state of the U.S. healthcare system and why there is such interest in its reform.

National Health Expenditures 2012 Highlights

The following document is a fact sheet from CMS that presents key facts and data on the nation's spending in the health sector. It is a good place to begin to understand the breath and scope of this spending.

In 2012 U.S. health care spending increased 3.7 percent to reach $2.8 trillion, or $8,915 per person, the fourth consecutive year of slow growth. The share of the economy devoted to health spending decreased from 17.3 percent in 2011 to 17.2 percent in 2012, as the Gross Domestic Product increased nearly one per-centage point faster than health care spending at 4.6 percent.

Health Spending by Type of Service or Product: Personal Healthcare

- **Hospital Care:** Hospital spending increased 4.9 percent to $882.3 billion in 2012 compared to 3.5-percent growth in 2011. The accelerated growth in 2012 was influenced by growth in both prices and non-price factors (which include the use and intensity of services). Growth in spending from Medicare, Medicaid, and private health insurance hospital spending all accelerated in 2012 compared to 2011.

- **Physician and Clinical Services:** Spending on physician and clinical services increased 4.6 percent in 2012 to $565.0 billion, from 4.1-percent growth in 2011. Although growth in prices slowed slightly in 2012, non-price factors such as the use and intensity of services increased faster in 2012. Growth in spending from private health insurance and Medicare, the two largest payers of physician and clinical services, experienced diverging trends in 2012. Private health insurance spending for physician and clinical services grew at a faster pace, while Medicare spending decelerated slightly in 2012.

- **Other Professional Services:** Spending for other professional services reached $76.4 billion in 2012, increasing 4.5 percent and about the same rate as in 2011 (4.6 percent). Spending in this category includes establishments of independent health practitioners (except physicians and dentists) that primarily provide services such as physical therapy, optometry, podiatry, and chiropractic medicine.

- **Dental Services:** Spending for dental services increased 3.0 percent in 2012 to $110.9 billion, faster than in 2011 when growth was 2.2 percent. Out-of-pocket spending for dental services (which accounted for 42 percent of all dental spending) increased 3.9 percent in 2012, following growth of 3.1 percent in 2011.

- **Other Health, Residential, and Personal Care Services:** Spending for other health, residential, and personal care services grew 4.5 percent in 2012 to $138.2 billion, an acceleration from growth of 3.3 percent in 2011. This category includes expenditures for medical services that are generally delivered by providers in non-traditional settings such as schools, community centers, the workplace, ambulance providers, and residential mental health and substance abuse facilities.

- **Home Healthcare:** Spending growth for freestanding home health care agencies accelerated in 2012, increasing 5.1 percent to $77.8 billion following growth of 4.1 percent in 2011. Medicare and Medicaid spending accounted for approximately 81 percent of total home health care spending in 2012. Medicare spending grew at a faster rate in 2012 while Medicaid spending slowed.

- **Nursing Care Facilities and Continuing Care Retirement Communities:** Spending for freestanding nursing care facilities and continuing care retirement communities increased 1.6 percent in 2012 to $151.5 billion, a deceleration from growth of 4.3 percent in 2011. The slower growth in 2012 was primarily due to a reduction in Medicare spending due to a one-time rate adjustment for skilled nursing facilities.

- **Prescription Drugs:** Retail prescription drug spending slowed in 2012, growing 0.4 percent to $263.3 billion, compared to 2.5-percent growth in 2011. The low growth in 2012 was driven largely by a slowdown in overall prices paid for retail prescription drugs, as numerous blockbuster drugs lost patent protection in late 2011 and 2012, and generic versions of those drugs became available.

- **Durable Medical Equipment:** Retail spending for durable medical equipment reached $41.3 billion in 2012, and increased 5.6 percent in 2012, the same rate of growth as in 2011. Spending in this category includes items such as contact lenses, eyeglasses and hearing aids.

- **Other Non-durable Medical Products:** Retail spending for other non-durable medical products, such as over-the-counter medicines, medical instruments, and surgical dressings grew 1.8 percent to $53.7 billion in 2012. This was a slower rate of growth than in 2011, when spending grew 3.0 percent.

Health Spending by Major Sources of Funds:

- **Medicare:** Medicare spending, which represented 20 percent of national health spending in 2012, grew 4.8 percent to $572.5 billion, a slight slowdown from growth of 5.0 percent in 2011. A one-time payment reduction to skilled nursing facilities in 2012, after a large increase in payments in

2011 due to implementation of a new payment system contributed to the slower growth.

- **Medicaid:** Total Medicaid spending grew 3.3 percent in 2012 to $421.2 billion, an acceleration from 2.4-percent growth in 2011. The relatively low annual rates of growth in Medicaid spending in 2011 and 2012 can be explained in part by slower enrollment growth tied to improved economic conditions and efforts by states to control health care costs. Federal Medicaid expenditures decreased 4.2 percent in 2012, while state and local Medicaid expenditures grew 15.0 percent—a result of the expiration of enhanced federal aid to states in the middle of 2011.

- **Private Health Insurance:** Overall, premiums reached $917.0 billion in 2012, and increased 3.2 percent, near the 3.4 percent growth in 2011. The net cost ratio for private health insurance—the difference between premiums and benefits as a share of premiums—was 12.0 percent in 2012 compared with 12.4 percent in 2011. Private health insurance enrollment increased 0.4 percent to 188.0 million in 2012, but still 9.4 million lower than in 2007.

- **Out-of-Pocket:** Out-of-pocket spending grew 3.8 percent in 2012 to $328.2 billion, an acceleration from growth of 3.5 percent in 2011, reflecting higher cost-sharing and increased enrollment in consumer-directed health plans.

Health Spending by Type of Sponsor[1]:

- In 2012, households accounted for the largest share of spending (28 percent), followed by the federal government

---

[1]Type of sponsor is defined as the entity that is ultimately responsible for financing the health care bill, such as a private business, household, or government. These sponsors pay insurance premiums, out-of-pocket costs, or finance health care through dedicated taxes or general revenues.

(26 percent), private businesses (21 percent), and state and local governments (18 percent).

- The federal government financed 26 percent of total health spending in 2012, a slight decrease from 27 percent in 2011. The reduction in the federal share reflects the expiration in June 2011of enhanced federal funding from the American Recovery and Reinvestment Act of 2009.
- The share of the health care bill financed by state and local governments increased from 17 percent in 2011 to 18 percent in 2012. This increased share of spending was due to states no longer receiving additional aid from the federal government in the form of enhanced matching rates.
- The remaining sponsors of health care maintained constant shares between 2011 and 2012—households (28 percent), private businesses (21 percent), and other private revenues (7 percent).

Source: https://www.cms.gov/Research-Statistics-Data-and -Systems/Statistics-Trends-and-Reports/NationalHealthExpend Data/Downloads/highlights.pdf

Data and Documents from Nongovernmental Sources

Figure 5.3 is a graphic presentation of data related to the states that have and have not taken advantage of the Medicaid expansion included in the Affordable Care Act. It was prepared by Family USA (FamiliesUSA.org). It not only shows what the 50 states decided to do but presents data on the impact on their health insurance coverage.

42 Changes to ObamaCare . . . So Far

The following document was published by the Galen Institute (http://www.galen.org/) and presents changes to the ACA that have been implemented since its passage. The version presented here was last updated on July 14, 2014.

By our count at the Galen Institute, more than 42 significant changes already have been made to ObamaCare: at least 24 that

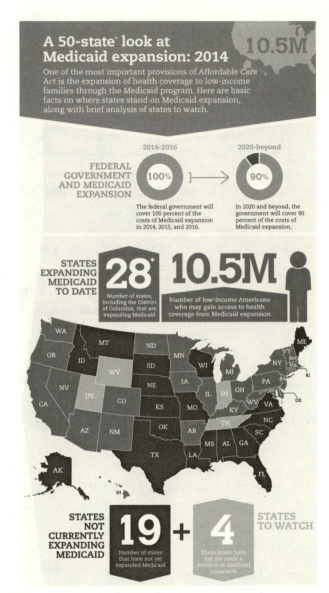

Figure 5.3a   A 50-State Look at Medicaid Expansion, 2014

Source: http://familiesusa.org/product/50-state-look-medicaid-expansion-2014.

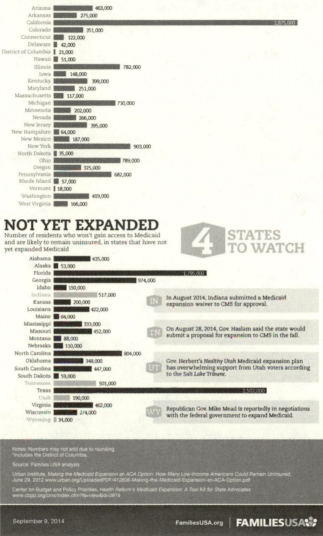

EXPANDING
Number of residents who may gain access to Medicaid, in states that will expand the program

Arizona	463,000
Arkansas	275,000
California	2,875,000
Colorado	351,000
Connecticut	122,000
Delaware	42,000
District of Columbia	21,000
Hawaii	51,000
Illinois	782,000
Iowa	148,000
Kentucky	399,000
Maryland	251,000
Massachusetts	117,000
Michigan	730,000
Minnesota	202,000
Nevada	266,000
New Jersey	395,000
New Hampshire	64,000
New Mexico	187,000
New York	903,000
North Dakota	35,000
Ohio	789,000
Oregon	325,000
Pennsylvania	682,000
Rhode Island	57,000
Vermont	18,000
Washington	419,000
West Virginia	166,000

NOT YET EXPANDED
Number of residents who won't gain access to Medicaid and are likely to remain uninsured, in states that have not yet expanded Medicaid

4 STATES TO WATCH

Alabama	435,000
Alaska	53,000
Florida	1,795,000
Georgia	974,000
Idaho	150,000
Indiana	517,000
Kansas	200,000
Louisiana	422,000
Maine	64,000
Mississippi	333,000
Missouri	452,000
Montana	88,000
Nebraska	110,000
North Carolina	804,000
Oklahoma	348,000
South Carolina	447,000
South Dakota	59,000
Tennessee	501,000
Texas	2,502,000
Utah	190,000
Virginia	462,000
Wisconsin	274,000
Wyoming	34,000

IN In August 2014, Indiana submitted a Medicaid expansion waiver to CMS for approval.

TN On August 28, 2014, Gov. Haslam said the state would submit a proposal for expansion to CMS in the fall.

UT Gov. Herbert's *Healthy Utah* Medicaid expansion plan has overwhelming support from Utah voters according to the *Salt Lake Tribune*.

WY Republican Gov. Mike Mead is reportedly in negotiations with the federal government to expand Medicaid.

Notes: Numbers may not add due to rounding.
*Includes the District of Columbia.

Source: Families USA analysis

Urban Institute, *Making the Medicaid Expansion an ACA Option: How Many Low-Income Americans Could Remain Uninsured*, June 29, 2012 www.urban.org/UploadedPDF/412606-Making-the-Medicaid-Expansion-an-ACA-Option.pdf

Center on Budget and Policy Priorities, *Health Reform's Medicaid Expansion: A Tool Kit for State Advocates* www.cbpp.org/cms/index.cfm?fa=view&id=3819

September 9, 2014   FamiliesUSA.org   **FAMILIESUSA**

Figure 5.3b   A 50-State Look at Medicaid Expansion, 2014

Source: http://familiesusa.org/product/50-state-look-medicaid-expansion-2014.

249

President Obama has made unilaterally, 16 that Congress has passed and the president has signed, and 2 by the Supreme Court.

CHANGES BY ADMINISTRATIVE ACTION

1. *Medicare Advantage patch*: The administration ordered an advance draw on funds from a Medicare bonus program in order to provide extra payments to Medicare Advantage plans, in an effort to temporarily forestall cuts in benefits and therefore delay early exodus of MA plans from the program. (April 19, 2011)

2. *Employee reporting*: The administration, contrary to the Obamacare legislation, instituted a one-year delay of the requirement that employers must report to their employees on their W-2 forms the full cost of their employer-provided health insurance. (January 1, 2012)

3. *Subsidies may flow through federal exchanges*: The IRS issued a rule that allows premium assistance tax credits to be available in federal exchanges although the law only specified that they would be available "through an Exchange established by the State under Section 1311." (May 23, 2012)

4. *Closing the high-risk pool*: The administration decided to halt enrollment in transitional federal high-risk pools created by the law, blocking coverage for an estimated 40,000 new applicants, citing a lack of funds. The administration had money from a fund under Secretary Sebelius's control to extend the pools, but instead used the money to pay for advertising for Obamacare enrollment and other purposes. (February 15, 2013)

5. *Doubling allowed deductibles*: Because some group health plans use more than one benefits administrator, plans are allowed to apply separate patient cost-sharing limits to different services, such as doctor/hospital and prescription drugs, allowing maximum out-of-pocket costs to be twice as high as the law intended. (February 20, 2013)

6. *Small businesses on hold*: The administration has said that the federal exchanges for small businesses will not be ready by the 2014 statutory deadline, and instead delayed until 2015 the provision of SHOP (Small-Employer Health Option Program) that requires the exchanges to offer a choice of qualified health plans. (March 11, 2013)

7. *Delaying a low-income plan*: The administration delayed implementation of the Basic Health Program until 2015. It would have provided more-affordable health coverage for certain low-income individuals not eligible for Medicaid. (March 22, 2013)

8. *Employer-mandate delay*: By an administrative action that's contrary to statutory language in the ACA, the reporting requirements for employers were delayed by one year. (July 2, 2013)

9. *Self-attestation*: Because of the difficulty of verifying income after the employer-reporting requirement was delayed, the administration decided it would allow "self-attestation" of income by applicants for health insurance in the exchanges. This was later partially retracted after congressional and public outcry over the likelihood of fraud. (July 15, 2013)

10. *Delaying the online SHOP exchange:* The administration first delayed for a month and later for a year until November 2014 the launch of the online insurance marketplace for small businesses. The exchange was originally scheduled to launch on October 1, 2013. (September 26, 2013) (November 27, 2013)

11. *Congressional opt-out*: The administration decided to offer employer contributions to members of Congress and their staffs when they purchase insurance on the exchanges created by the ACA, a subsidy the law doesn't provide. (September 30, 2013)

12. *Delaying the individual mandate*: The administration changed the deadline for the individual mandate, by declaring that customers who have purchased insurance by March 31, 2014 will avoid the tax penalty. Previously, they

would have had to purchase a plan by mid-February. (October 23, 2013)

13. *Insurance companies may offer canceled plans:* The administration announced that insurance companies may reoffer plans that previous regulations forced them to cancel. (November 14, 2013)

14. *Exempting unions from reinsurance fee:* The administration gave unions an exemption from the reinsurance fee (one of ObamaCare's many new taxes). To make up for this exemption, non-exempt plans will have to pay a higher fee, which will likely be passed onto consumers in the form of higher premiums and deductibles. (December 2, 2013)

15. *Extending Preexisting Condition Insurance Plan:* The administration extended the federal high risk pool until January 31, 2014 and again until March 15, 2014 to prevent a coverage gap for the most vulnerable. The plans were scheduled to expire on December 31, but were extended because it has been impossible for some to sign up for new coverage on healthcare.gov. (December 12, 2013) (January 14, 2014)

16. *Expanding hardship waiver to those with canceled plans:* The administration expanded the hardship waiver, which excludes people from the individual mandate and allows some to purchase catastrophic health insurance, to people who have had their plans canceled because of ObamaCare regulations. The administration later extended this waiver until October 1, 2016. (December 19, 2013) (March 5, 2014)

17. *Equal employer coverage delayed:* Tax officials will not be enforcing in 2014 the mandate requiring employers to offer equal coverage to all their employees. This provision of the law was supposed to go into effect in 2010, but IRS officials have "yet to issue regulations for employers to follow." (January 18, 2013)

18. *Employer-mandate delayed again:* The administration delayed for an additional year provisions of the employer mandate, postponing enforcement of the requirement for medium-size employers until 2016 and relaxing some

requirements for larger employers. Businesses with 100 or more employees must offer coverage to 70% of their full-time employees in 2015 and 95% in 2016 and beyond. (February 10, 2014)

19. *Extending subsidies to non-exchange plans*: The administration released a bulletin through CMS extending subsidies to individuals who purchased health insurance plans outside of the federal or state exchanges. The bulletin also requires retroactive coverage and subsidies for individuals from the date they applied on the marketplace rather than the date they actually enrolled in a plan. (February 27, 2014)

20. *Non-compliant health plans get two year extension*: The administration pushed back the deadline by two years that requires health insurers to cancel plans that are not compliant with ObamaCare's mandates. These "illegal" plans may now be offered until 2017. This extension will prevent a wave cancellation notices from going out before the 2014 midterm elections. (March 5, 2014)

21. *Delaying the sign-up deadline*: The administration delayed until mid-April the March 31 deadline to sign up for insurance. Applicants simply need to check a box on their application to qualify for this extended sign-up period. (March 26, 2014)

22. *Canceling Medicare Advantage cuts:* The administration canceled scheduled cuts to Medicare Advantage. The ACA calls for $200 billion in cuts to Medicare Advantage over 10 years. (April 7, 2014)

23. *More Funds for Insurer Bailout:* The administration said it will supplement risk corridor payments to health insurance plans with "other sources of funding" if the higher risk profile of enrollees means the plans would lose money. (May 16, 2014)

24. *Exempting U.S. territories:* Despite earlier administration claims that "HHS is not authorized to choose which provisions [of the ACA] might apply to the territories," HHS waived six major requirements—such as guaranteed issue,

community rating, and essential benefit mandates—that were causing serious disruption to health insurance markets. (July 18, 2014)

25. *Failure to enforce abortion restrictions*: A GAO report found that many exchange insurance plans don't separate charges for abortion services as required by the ACA, showing that the administration is not enforcing the law. In 2014, abortions were being financed with taxpayer funds in more than 1,000 exchange plans. (Sept. 16, 2014)

26. *Risk Corridor coverage*: The Obama administration plans to illegally distribute risk corridor payments to insurers, despite studies by both the Congressional Research Service and the GAO saying a congressional appropriation is required before federal agencies can make the payments. (Sept. 30, 2014)

27. *Transparency of coverage*: CMS delays statutory requirements on insurance companies to disclose data on the number of people enrolled, disenrollment, number of claims denied, costs to consumers of certain services, etc. (Oct. 20, 2014)

28. *Bay State Bailout*: More than 300,000 people in Massachusetts gained temporary Medicaid coverage in 2014 without any verification of their eligibility, with the Obama and Patrick administrations using a taxpayer-funded bailout to mask the failure of the commonwealth's disastrously malfunctioning website. (January 2014)

CHANGES BY CONGRESS, SIGNED BY PRESIDENT OBAMA:

29. *Military benefits*: Congress clarified that plans provided by TRICARE, the military's health-insurance program, constitutes minimal essential health-care coverage as required by the ACA; its benefits and plans wouldn't normally meet ACA requirements. (April 26, 2010)

30. *VA benefits*: Congress also clarified that health care provided by the Department of Veterans Affairs constitutes minimum essential health-care coverage as required by the ACA. (May 27, 2010)

31. *Drug-price clarification*: Congress modified the definition of average manufacturer price (AMP) to include inhalation, infusion, implanted, or injectable drugs that are not generally dispensed through a retail pharmacy. (August 10, 2010)

32. *Doc-fix tax*: Congress modified the amount of premium tax credits that individuals would have to repay if they are over-allotted, an action designed to help offset the costs of the postponement of cuts in Medicare physician payments called for in the ACA. (December 15, 2010)

33. *Extending the adoption credit*: Congress extended the nonrefundable adoption tax credit, which happened to be included in the ACA, through tax year 2012. (December 17, 2010)

34. *TRICARE for adult children*: Congress extended TRICARE coverage to dependent adult children up to age 26 when it had previously only covered those up to the age of 21—though beneficiaries still have to pay premiums for them. (January 7, 2011)

35. *1099 repealed*: Congress repealed the paperwork ("1099") mandate that would have required businesses to report to the IRS all of their transactions with vendors totaling $600 or more in a year. (April 14, 2011)

36. *No free-choice vouchers*: Congress repealed a program, supported by Senator Ron Wyden (D., Ore.) that would have allowed "free-choice vouchers," that the *Hill* warned "could lead young, healthy workers to opt out" of their employer plans, "driving up costs for everybody else." The same law barred additional funds for the IRS to hire new agents to enforce the health-care law. (April 15, 2011)

37. *No Medicaid for well-to-do seniors*: Congress saved taxpayers $13 billion by changing how the eligibility for certain

programs is calculated under Obamacare. Without the change, a couple earning as much as much as $64,000 would still have been able to qualify for Medicaid. (November 21, 2011)

38. *CO-OPs, IPAB, IRS defunded*: Congress made further cuts to agencies implementing Obamacare. It trimmed another $400 million off the CO-OP program, cut another $305 million from the IRS to hamper its ability to enforce the law's tax hikes and mandates, and rescinded $10 million in funding for the controversial Independent Payment Advisory Board. (December 23, 2011)

39. *Slush-fund savings*: Congress slashed another $11.6 billion from the Prevention and Public Health slush fund and $2.5 billion from Obamacare's "Louisiana Purchase." (February 22, 2012)

40. *Less cash for Louisiana*: One of the tricks used to get Obamacare through the Senate was the special "Louisiana Purchase" deal for the state's Democratic senator, Mary Landrieu. Congress saved another $670 million by rescinding additional funds from this bargain. (July 6, 2012)

41. *CLASS Act eliminated*: Congress repealed the unsustainable CLASS (Community Living Assistance Services and Supports) program of government-subsidized long-term-care insurance, which even the Democratic chairman of the Senate Finance Committee dubbed a "Ponzi scheme of the first order." (January 2, 2013)

42. *Cutting CO-OPs*: Congress cut $2.2 billion from the "Consumer Operated and Oriented Plan" (CO-OP), which some saw as a stealth public option, blocking creation of government-subsidized co-op insurance programs in about half the states. Early reports showed many co-ops, which had received federal loans, had run into serious financial trouble. (January 2, 2013)

43. *Trimming the Medicare trust-fund transfer*: Congress rescinded $200 million of the $500 million scheduled to be taken from the Medicare Part A and Part B trust funds and

sent to the Community-Based Care Transition Program established and funded by the ACA. (March 26, 2013)

44. *Eliminating caps on deductibles for small group plans:* Congress eliminated the cap on deductibles for small group plans as part of the SGR "doc fix." This change gives small businesses the freedom to offer high deductible plans that may be paired with a Health Savings Account. (April 1, 2014)

45. Making the risk corridor program budget neutral. The Consolidated and Further Continuing Appropriations Act of 2015 provides that CMS may not transfer funds from other accounts to pay for the risk corridor program. Expenditures cannot exceed the funds collected in 2014, blocking CMS from making multi-year calculations. (December 16, 2014).

CHANGES BY THE SUPREME COURT:

46. *Medicare expansion made voluntary:* The court ruled it had to be voluntary, rather than mandatory, for states to expand Medicaid eligibility to people with incomes up to 138 percent of the federal poverty level, by ruling that the federal government couldn't halt funds for existing state Medicaid programs if they chose not to expand the program.

47. *The individual mandate made a tax:* The court determined that violating the mandate that Americans must purchase government-approved health insurance would only result in individuals' paying a "tax," making it, legally speaking, optional for people to comply.

This list was originally published on Galen.org and has been published on National Review Online. It was updated to 29 changes on December 10, 2013.

December 13, 2013 UPDATE: 30 changes (PCIP extension)

December 19, 2013 UPDATE: 31 changes (Hardship waiver)

January 14, 2014 UPDATE: 32 changes (Union reinsurance fee exemption)

January 14, 2014 UPDATE: (PCIP extended again)

January 21, 2014 UPDATE: 33 changes (Equal employer coverage delay)

February 3, 2014 UPDATE: 34 changes (Subsidies may flow through federal exchanges) (List is now ordered chronologically)

February 10, 2014 UPDATE: 35 changes (Second employer mandate delay)

March 5, 2014 UPDATE: 36 changes (Subsidies extended outside of exchanges)

March 5, 2014 UPDATE: 37 changes (Consumers can keep non-compliant plans until 2017)

March 26, 2014 UPDATE: 38 changes (Sign-up deadline delayed)

April 7, 2014 UPDATE: 39 changes (Small group deductible cap eliminated-passed by Congress and signed into law)

April 8, 2014 UPDATE: 40 changes (Cuts to Medicare Advantage in 2015 canceled)

May 22, 2014 UPDATE: 41 changes (More funds for insurer bailout)

July 18, 2014 UPDATE: 42 changes (Exempting U.S. Territories)

December 26, 2014 UPDATE: 46 changes (Failure to enforce abortion restrictions; Risk Corridor coverage; Transparency of coverage; Bay State Bailout)

January 7, 2015 UPDATE: 47 changes (Making the risk corridor program budget neutral)

Source: Tyler Hartsfield and Grace-Marie Turner, http://www.galen.org/newsletters/changes-to-obamacare-so-far/. Used by permission of the Galen Institute.

Figure 5.4 reviews the benefits and costs of the Affordable Care Act for consumers. The fact sheet is presented by Time for Affordability, an educational campaign sponsored by health insurance companies.

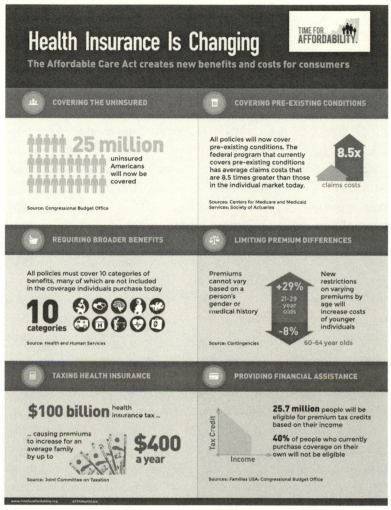

Figure 5.4   Health Insurance Is Changing: The Affordable Care Act Creates New Benefits and Costs for Consumers

Source: http://timeforaffordability.org/wp-content/uploads/2013/06/timeforaffordability -factsheet.png.

The ACA: Some Unpleasant Welfare Arithmetic

The following document presents a conservative view on the impact of the Affordable Care Act. It was produced by the Cato Institute, a conservative think tank described on its website (http://www .cato.org/about) as "a public policy research organization—a think

tank—dedicated to the principles of individual liberty, limited government, free markets and peace."

The Affordable Care Act (ACA) presents employers and potential employees with a variety of new rewards and penalties. These are, in part, exactly what the law intended: by penalizing potential employees for not purchasing health insurance, and employers for not providing it, the law aims to increase the fraction of the population with health insurance. Yet these same rewards and penalties have additional effects, including on the incentive to work; Mulligan (2014), for example, suggests that the ACA may reduce employment by 3 percent on average and have a range of positive and negative effects on average hours worked.

In the work summarized here, I quantify the number of people who will have essentially no short-term financial reward from working more than 29 hours, since this would either render them ineligible for the ACA's assistance or increase the penalties that may be owed by their employer. This is the first paper to show that the ACA will put millions of workers in the economically extreme situation of having zero short-term financial reward (or less) to working full-time rather than part-time.

In economics jargon, this means the ACA creates marginal tax rates on labor income that exceed 100 percent. Even when helping people who are out of work or who otherwise have low incomes is a primary policy motivation, and even if labor supply does not respond much to the after-tax wage, labor income tax rates that equal or exceed 100 percent are bad policy because they discourage work effort without raising any revenue.

From a strictly predictive perspective, economists expect that full-time employment rates will be low, if not zero, in groups of people who are aware that they receive no financial reward from working full-time (defined here to be working at least 30 hours per week).

Two separate ACA provisions can fully eliminate the reward to full-time work. The first, which is scheduled to be in full force in 2016, pertains to full-time employees of firms that do not offer health insurance: by cutting weekly work hours to 29, they save their employer the annual salary equivalent of more than $3,000, or, they save their employers the threat of even larger penalties. Women workers, young workers, and persons already working 30–35 hour schedules are especially likely to have their short-term financial reward to full-time work erased by the ACA. By my estimates, three to four million workers overall will fall victim to this penalty provision.

The second provision pertains to full-time employees at firms that do offer health insurance. Over 60 million workers obtain health insurance from their employer, not including workers who obtain health insurance from a family member's employer. About half of them (26 million) are in families between 100 and 400 percent of the poverty line and therefore satisfy the income criteria for exchange subsidies. And 11 million of those are unmarried—so by definition cannot be covered by a spouse's plan—and another 8 million of the married have a spouse that does not work or otherwise cannot obtain coverage through a spouse.

In other words, almost 20 million workers are ineligible for exchange subsidies solely because their employer offers coverage to full-time employees: these are the workers subject to the ACA's implicit full-time employment tax (FTET). A 29-hour work schedule, on the other hand, would make them eligible for subsidies without creating any penalty for the employer.

In about four million cases (of the 20 million facing an implicit FTET of some magnitude), the dollar amount of subsidy gain can exceed the after-tax income that is earned for working beyond 29 hours per week. A distinguishing feature of almost 90 percent of these workers is that their family incomes are below 250 percent of the federal poverty line. The four million disproportionately consist of working unmarried household heads because, as noted, unmarried heads are especially likely to be ineligible for exchange subsidies solely because their employer is offering coverage to full-time employees.

Older (but not elderly) workers are also disproportionately represented among those facing an implicit FTET rate of 100+ percent, since older workers are more likely to have employer-sponsored insurance and are more expensive to insure. The 100+ percent FTET from the employer penalty has the opposite age pattern, which means there may be little age pattern for the propensity to face one of the 100+ percent FTETs.

The prevalence of 100+ percent FTETs is an important indicator of its effects on incentives to work, but it is not the only one. There are other ways to avoid the FTET, such as working more hours per week for fewer weeks of the year. If employers are unwilling or unable to adjust work schedules, the FTET may affect the equilibrium relationship between hours and earnings (i.e., compensating differences) rather than changing the distribution of hours. At the other extreme, employers may be able to substantially adjust measured work hours without changing the actual work that is done (e.g., require employees to "punch out" during break periods, and then adjust their hourly wage so that weekly earnings are the same), in which case the ACA will reduce the measured hours for quite a large number of workers.

In effect, millions of workers are becoming eligible for fully federally funded paid days off, akin to the sick leave policies in Western European countries. Because the Western European data suggest that paid sick days really do result in fewer days at work (Lusinyan 2007), we should expect the act's FTETs to reduce days worked as well, at least for the segments of the workforce that do not avoid the ACA's taxes in other ways.

These effects of the ACA are only part of its impact; people who believe government should provide health insurance for everyone may regard these costs—the disincentive effects discussed here and elsewhere—as worth paying.

But everyone should recognize that the ACA's costs are likely to exceed the budgetary expenditure.

NOTE

This Research Brief is based on Casey B. Mulligan, "The ACA: Some Unpleasant Welfare Arithmetic," National Bureau of Economics Working Paper No. 20020, available at http://www .nber.org/papers/w20020. All works cited are provided there.

Source: Casey B. Mulligan, "The ACA: Some Unpleasant Welfare Arithmetic," Research Briefs in Economic Policy, June 2014, No. 3. The Cato Institute. Available online at http://www.cato.org/publications/research-briefs-economic-policy/aca-some-unpleasant-welfare-arithmetic

Cutting Healthcare Costs: Leading Experts Propose Bold Solutions

The following document presents recommendations from healthcare cost experts on how to cut healthcare costs, collected by the Center for American Progress.

The Affordable Care Act is the most far-reaching effort to contain health care costs to date. The new law includes an array of reforms to the way health care is paid for and delivered—reforms that reward the value and quality of care, not just the quantity of care. These signals to health care providers are already catalyzing change throughout the health care system.

But health care costs remain a major challenge. National health spending is projected to continue to grow faster than the economy, increasing from 18 percent of the economy to about 25 percent by 2037. Even with the new law, federal health spending is projected to increase from 25 percent of total federal spending to about 40 percent by 2037.

These trends could squeeze out critical investments in education and infrastructure, contribute to unsustainable debt levels, and constrain wage increases for middle-class workers. The Center for American Progress convened leading health policy experts—including current and former federal and state officials, executives of health insurers and hospital systems, physicians, and economists—to develop bold and innovative solutions to contain health care costs. These are their recommendations.

A systemic approach

Reforms that simply shift federal spending to individuals, employers, and states fail to address the problem—and would ultimately lead many people to forgo necessary care. The only sustainable solution is to control overall growth in health care costs. The following solutions are designed to reduce overall health care spending for both public and private payers.

Promote privately negotiated payment rates within global spending targets

Payers and providers should negotiate payment rates that would be binding for all payers and providers in a state. The privately negotiated rates would have to fit within a global spending target for both public and private payers in the state.

Accelerate use of alternatives to fee-for-service payment

Instead of paying a fee for each service, physicians and hospitals should receive a fixed amount for a bundle of services (also called bundled payments) or for all the care a patient needs (known as global payments). Payers must accelerate use of such alternative payment methods. Within 10 years, Medicare and Medicaid should base at least 75 percent of payments on alternatives to fee-for-service payment.

Use competitive bidding for all health care commodities

Instead of the government setting prices for health care commodities, manufacturers and suppliers should compete to offer the lowest price. Medicare should immediately expand such competitive bidding nationwide—and extend it to medical devices, laboratory tests, and all other commodities. Medicare's market-based prices should then be extended to all federal health programs.

Require exchanges to offer tiered plans

Tiered insurance plans designate a tier of providers with high quality and low costs, and reduce cost-sharing for patients who choose these high-value providers. Exchanges—marketplaces for insurance created by the health reform law—should offer at least one tiered plan with a premium discount of 10 percent or more.

Require all exchanges to be active purchasers

Both federal and state exchanges should engage in "active purchasing"—leveraging their bargaining power to secure the best premium rates and promote reforms that provide better care at lower cost.

Simplify administrative systems

Payers and providers should electronically exchange eligibility, claims, and other administrative information. A taskforce of payers and providers should set binding compliance targets, monitor use rates, and have broad authority to implement additional measures to achieve systemwide savings of $30 billion a year.

Require full price transparency

It is common sense that consumers should know how much something costs before treatment. All private insurers and states should provide price information that reflects negotiated discounts with specific providers.

Empower nonphysician providers

Restrictive state laws prevent nonphysician providers such as advanced-practice nurses from practicing to the full extent of their training. Making greater use of these providers would expand the workforce supply, which would increase competition and lower prices.

Prohibit physician self-referrals

Many studies show that when physicians refer patients to facilities in which they have a financial interest, they drive up costs and may negatively affect the quality of care. Such physician self-referrals should be strictly prohibited.

Leverage the Federal Employees Health Benefits Program to drive reform

The program should require participating health plans to reform their payment and delivery systems—including a transition to alternatives to fee-for-service payment.

Reduce the costs of defensive medicine

Under a "safe harbor," physicians would be presumed to have no liability for medical malpractice if they adhere to evidence-based clinical practice guidelines and use qualified health information technology.

What the experts are saying

"The Affordable Care Act was the first generation of reforms to tackle cost growth. These ideas are the next generation. They provide a roadmap to make America more competitive in the global economy because as we lower health care costs, we lower the costs of hiring new workers."

—Neera Tanden, J.D., President, Center for American Progress

"Ever rising health care costs reduce middle-class families' take-home pay and threaten America's standing in the world. These proposals would build on the health reform law to dramatically improve our health care system. As Congress looks to cut the budget—and health care spending in particular—these proposals offer a roadmap that can transform the system and produce substantial savings."

—Ezekiel Emanuel, M.D., Ph.D., Senior Fellow, Center for American Progress

"Rising health care costs pose a direct threat to workers' take-home pay, the federal budget, and state government finances. The key question is how we can continue the recent deceleration in health costs. These ideas—from expanding bundled payments to an innovative malpractice reform—represent a promising approach to moving toward a higher-value health care system."

—Peter Orszag, vice president, Citigroup, Inc.; former director, Office of Management and Budget

"It is both important and completely feasible to reduce health care costs without any harm whatsoever to patients. Indeed, improvement of care is by far the best strategy for making care affordable. These ideas offer many helpful steps toward that goal."

—Donald Berwick, Senior Fellow, Center for American Progress and Harvard Medical School; former administrator, Centers for Medicare and Medicaid Services

"This set of proposals offers a real way forward, away from the stale debates that have consumed so much of policymaking."

—David Cutler, Senior Fellow, Center for American Progress; Otto Eckstein professor of applied economics, Harvard University

"These principles are a strong foundation that can set the U.S. health care system on a path of sustainable growth. Businesses in particular have an immediate need for value and innovation so that we have a health care delivery system that rewards quality and efficiency."

—Sally Welborn, senior vice president, benefits, Walmart Stores Inc.

"Safely holding health industry income growth to what average Americans can afford and taxpayers are willing to pay has vexed politicians and policymakers for decades. As illustrated by this thought piece, success will likely require leverage from the market, from regulators, and from health industry leaders."

—Dr. Arnold Milstein, M.D., professor of medicine, Stanford University; medical director, Pacific Business Group on Health

"The cut and shift approach advocated by many is fundamentally flawed. These ideas represent a better approach that will protect access to necessary care. Most important, they will put us on the path toward an actual health care system."

—Former Sen. Tom Daschle, Distinguished Senior Fellow, Center for American Progress; senior policy advisor, DLA Piper

"The passage of the Affordable Care Act was not the last step in the push to reform our health care system. If Team USA is to succeed in the 21st century, we need to continue to reform the health care sector to lower costs and increase efficiency, while also raising the quality of care. Health care reform, as detailed in this report, can be the engine that puts our country back on track."

—Andy Stern, senior fellow, Columbia University; former president, Service Employees International Union

"Achieving the full promise of the Affordable Care Act requires that we take concrete steps on multiple fronts to give patients and their physicians opportunities to make higher-value health care choices. This proposal offers a set of evidence-based, high-impact, feasible policies that will put the health care system on a more sustainable path."

—Meredith Rosenthal, Ph.D., professor of health economics and policy, Harvard School of Public Health

"These ideas represent a look down the field to a health care system that controls costs and improves health at the same time."

—Joshua Sharfstein, secretary of health and mental hygiene, state of Maryland

"These ideas represent a huge next step for improving our health system—they will spur innovation, new ways of thinking, and new investment. As a result, new companies will be formed, new jobs will be created, and new technology will be invented that will make our health system more reliable and the marketplace more competitive. These policies make good policy sense, fiscal sense, and business sense."

—Bob Kocher, partner, Venrock; former senior advisor, National Economic Council

"We need to move more quickly toward a health care system that all Americans can afford, while increasing the quality of our lives. These ideas will help drive us down that path."

—Stephen Shortell, dean, University of California, Berkeley, School of Public Health

Source: Center for American Progress, August 2, 2012. Available online at http://cdn.americanprogress.org/wp-content/uploads/issues/2012/08/pdf/nejm_fact_sheet.pdf. This material was created by the Center for American Progress (www.americanprogress.org).

The Affordable Care Act's Lower-Than-Projected Premiums Will Save $190 Billion

The following report, also produced by the Center for American Progress, reviews health insurance premium costs after the first year's enrollment in Affordable Health Care Markets.

The Affordable Care Act is already working: Intense price competition among health plans in the marketplaces for individuals has lowered premiums below projected levels. As a result of these lower premiums, the federal government will save about $190 billion over the next 10 years, according to our estimates. These savings will boost the health law's amount of deficit reduction by 174 percent and represent about 40 percent of the health care savings proposed by the National Commission on Fiscal Responsibility and Reform—commonly known as the Simpson-Bowles commission—in 2010.

Moreover, we estimate that lower premiums will lower the number of uninsured even further, by an additional 700,000 people, even as the number of individuals who receive tax credits will decline because insurance is more affordable.

In short, the Affordable Care Act is working even better than expected, producing more coverage for much less money.

Marketplace plans and tax credits

Under the Affordable Care Act, marketplaces that offer health plans to individuals are now open in every state. The federal government is operating marketplaces in 36 states, and 14 states and the District of Columbia are operating their own marketplaces. Marketplace plans offer five levels of coverage—catastrophic, bronze, silver, gold, and platinum—ranging from less generous to more generous.

Individuals with family income from one to four times the federal poverty level (about $26,000 to $94,000 for a family of four)—and who are not eligible for other qualified coverage—are eligible for tax credits to help cover the cost of a plan. The tax credit caps the amount an individual must pay for the second-lowest-cost silver plan at a certain percentage of family income, ranging from 2 percent of income at the poverty level to 9.5 percent of income at four times the poverty level.

Price competition in the marketplaces

When the nonpartisan Congressional Budget Office, or CBO, projected premiums under the Affordable Care Act before its enactment, it theorized that increased competition would lower premiums in the individual market—but only slightly. In CBO's view, marketplaces that organize the market—making it easier for consumers to compare choices—would encourage plans to keep premiums low to attract consumers.

CBO's theory has turned out to be right in reality—only more so.

In an analysis of plans offered in the marketplaces, the McKinsey Center for U.S. Health System Reform found that new entrants into the market make up 26 percent of all insurers. These new entrants are introducing competitive pressures into the individual market. The McKinsey analysis found that new entrants tend to price their plans lower than the median premiums in their market.

Moreover, in a preliminary analysis of plans offered in 18 areas, the Kaiser Family Foundation found that premiums are lower than CBO's projected premiums in 15 of those areas.

In March 2012, CBO projected an average family premium for the second-lowest-cost silver plan in 2016. This projection is equivalent to an average individual premium in 2014 of $4,700. The *actual* average premium for the second-lowest-cost silver plan in 2014 turned out to be $3,936—16 percent lower than projected.

CBO's projected premium levels

In March 2012, CBO projected an average family premium for the second-lowest-cost silver plan of $15,400 in 2016. This family premium is equivalent to an individual premium of $5,700 in 2016. CBO projected that private insurance premiums would increase by 5.5 percent per year from 2014 to 2016, so its estimate for 2014 would be lower by that amount. In addition, the Affordable Care Act covers the cost of high-risk enrollees through 2016, but it provides greater relief in 2014 than in 2016. This reinsurance will lower premiums by more in 2014 than in 2016. Taking the estimate of $5,700 in 2016, trending it backward by 5.5 percent per year, and accounting for greater reinsurance in 2014 yields an estimate of $4,700 in 2014.

Impact on costs and coverage

Premiums for the second-lowest-cost silver plan are important because tax credits for individuals are based on the cost of that plan. If premiums for that plan are lower, then the cost of tax credits will also be lower.

Consider a typical individual making $30,000 a year. That individual's premium contribution would be capped at 8.37 percent of income, or $2,512. If the premium for the second-lowest-cost silver plan is $4,700, then the tax credit would be the difference between this premium and the individual's contribution, or $2,188. But if the premium for the second-lowest-cost silver plan turns out to be only $3,936, then the tax credit would be $1,424.

We estimate that a 16 percent reduction in premiums will lower the total cost of tax credits by about 21 percent. As the example above illustrates, the percentage reduction in the tax credit will often be much greater than the percentage reduction in the premium. Because the amount that individuals pay is fixed at a percentage of income, a reduction in premiums will result in a proportionally larger reduction in government spending.

In its May 2013 baseline, CBO projected that the tax credits would cost $920 billion through 2023. But CBO made this projection before data on actual premium rates became available. A 16 percent reduction in premiums will lower this cost by about 21 percent, or about $190 billion.

Another result of the reduction in premiums is that more individuals will take up coverage because it is even more affordable. We estimate that a 16 percent reduction in premiums will lower the number of uninsured by an additional 2.8 percent. Because CBO had projected a decline in the number of uninsured of 25 million by 2023, this means that an additional 700,000 people will gain coverage. (See Methodology for more information on our estimates.)

$190 billion in context

When it was enacted, the Affordable Care Act was already fully paid for and projected to lower the federal budget deficit. In its most recent estimate, CBO projected that the law would lower the deficit by $109 billion over the next 10 years. Our estimated $190 billion in savings will increase that deficit reduction by 174 percent to almost $300 billion.

Recent long-term debt-reduction plans have proposed substantial health care savings in combination with additional tax revenue. The Simpson-Bowles commission, for example, proposed $487 billion in health care savings. And in the last "grand bargain" offer that President Barack Obama made to House Speaker John Boehner (R-OH) in December 2012, he proposed about $400 billion in health care savings.

Our estimated $190 billion in savings represents a sizable share of these proposals' health care savings—about 40 percent of the Simpson-Bowles plan's savings and almost half of the president's proposed savings.

Conclusion

In the spring, CBO will update its baseline projection of the Affordable Care Act. When it does, the agency will take into account the actual experience of premium rates for plans offered in the marketplaces in 2014—which are significantly lower than projected. We estimate that the savings to the federal government will be about $190 billion over the next 10 years. This is an important early indication that the

Affordable Care Act is working even better than expected to lower health care spending and federal deficits.

Source: Topher Spiro and Johnathan Gruber, October 23, 2013, Center for American Progress. Available online at http://www.americanprogress.org/issues/healthcare/report/2013/10/23/77537/the-affordable-care-acts-lower-than-projected-premiums-will-save-190-billion/. This material was created by the Center for American Progress (www.american progress.org).

The report *Gaining Ground: Americans' Health Insurance Coverage and Access to Care after the Affordable Care Act's First Open Enrollment Period* presents information on the impact of the first year of open enrollement in the Affordable Care Act on the number of uninsured Americans. Figures 5.5 and 5.6 are 2 of 18 figures in the report, which breaks down the numbers by income, race, and state resided in as well as the impact on this enrollment.

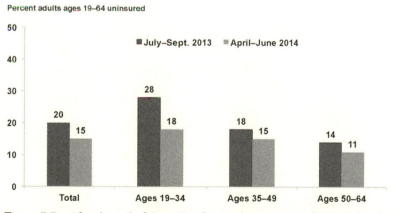

Figure 5.5 After the end of Open Enrollment, the percentage of U.S. adults who are uninsured declined from 20 percent to 15 percent, or by 9.5 million; young adults experienced the largest decline among all adult age groups.

Source: Collins, Sara R., Petra W. Rasmussen, Michelle M. Doty, *Gaining Ground: Americans' Health Insurance Coverage and Access to Care after the Affordable Care Act's First Open Enrollment Period*, The Commonwealth Fund, July 2014. Available online at http://www.commonwealthfund.org/~/media/files/publications/issue-brief/2014/jul/pdf_collins_gaining_ground_tracking_survey_april_june_2014_exhibits.pdf. Used by permission of The Commonwealth Fund.

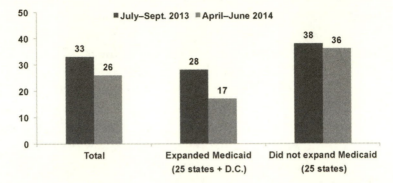

Percent adults ages 19–64 with incomes below 100 percent of poverty who were uninsured

Note: States were coded as expanding their Medicaid program if they began enrolling individuals in April or earlier. These states include AR, AZ, CA, CO, CT, DE, HI, IA, IL, KY, MA, MD, MI, MN, ND, NJ, NM, NV, NY, OH, OR, RI, VT, WA, WV, and the District of Columbia. All other states were coded as not expanding.

Figure 5.6   The percent of uninsured adults with incomes under 100 percent of poverty fell sharpley in states that expanded Medicaid; more than a third of poor adults remained uninsured in states that did not expand Medicaid.

Source: Collins, Sara R., Petra W. Rasmussen, Michelle M. Doty, *Gaining Ground: Americans' Health Insurance Coverage and Access to Care after the Affordable Care Act's First Open Enrollment Period*, The Commonwealth Fund, July 2014. Available online at http://www.commonwealthfund.org/~/media/files/publications/issue-brief/2014/jul/pdf_collins_gaining_ground_tracking_survey_april_june_2014_exhibits.pdf. Used by permission of The Commonwealth Fund.

NO MANDATE
NO ONE POLICY
FITS ALL
OBAMACARE
DYING / DEAD

Books and Reports on Health Reform

Alford, Robert R. (1975). *Health Care Politics: Ideological and Interest Group Barriers to Reform.* Chicago: University of Chicago Press.

This book incorporates the development of categories of interest groups and how they impact healthcare politics. Alford discusses three different approaches to reform of healthcare in the United States: market reforms, bureaucratic reforms and the structural interest approach. The first two are incremental approaches, while the third is a more comprehensive reform approach.

Altman, Stuart, and David Schactman. (2011). *Power, Politics, and Universal Health Care: The Inside Story of a Century-Long Battle.* Amherst, NY: Prometheus.

This book describes the sometimes haphazard, piece-by-piece construction of the nation's healthcare system, from the early efforts of Franklin Roosevelt and Harry Truman to the later additions of Ronald Reagan and George W. Bush. In each case, the authors examine the factors that led to success or failure, often by illuminating little-known

Healthcare reform protestors decry "Obamacare" outside the Supreme Court building in Washington, D.C., on June 28, 2012. (Richard Gunion/Dreamstime.com)

political maneuvers that brought about immense shifts in policy or thwarted herculean efforts at reform.

Blumenthal, David, and James Morone. (2010). *The Heart of Power: Health and Politics in the Oval Office.* Berekley: University of California Press.
> This book relates the 75-year history of presidential efforts to reform the U.S. healthcare system.

Budrys, Grace. (2005). *Our Unsystematic Health Care System,* 2nd ed. Lanham, MD: Rowman & Littlefield.
> This book provides an examination of the healthcare system as a social institution. It covers topics such as hospitals and healthcare organizations, the division of labor in healthcare organizations, health insurance issues, healthcare cost issues, and healthcare reform issues. It also includes some comparative material with healthcare systems in other countries.

Cohn, Jonathan. (2007). *Sick: The Untold Story of America's Health Care Crisis and the People Who Pay the Price.* New York: Harper Collins.
> This book follows more of a reporting style in which Jonathan Cole travels across the United States and reports on problems people have accessing healthcare services of all types. The book concludes in Washington, DC, and discusses issues within the medical industry and especially the healthcare insurance industry that have led to the problems Cole found in the United States.

Davidson, Stephen M. (2010). *Still Broken: Understanding the U.S. Health Care System.* Stanford, CA: Stanford Business Books.
> This book looks at: why the healthcare system is so important for us, how it really works, what caused the problems that have persisted for decades (and will continue under a new law), how we can solve them, and why we have failed to surmount these problems in the past. It describes six

elements that are critical to a successful reform plan and how various compromises related to those elements can affect what a new law will produce (taken from book's preface).

Emanuel, Ezekiel. (2008). *Healthcare Guaranteed: A Simple, Secure Solution for America.* New York: Public Affairs.

Emmanuel is a researcher with the National Institutes of Health, although this book represents his own opinions as a scholar, not official opinions of the National Institutes of Health. He argues that the cost of healthcare in the United States is skyrocketing, but American has mediocre health outcomes and substantial numbers of people without health insurance. Emmanuel proposes a program called the Guaranteed HealthCare Access Plan that would be a comprehensive reform plan to ensure coverage for all Americans by replacing employer healthcare with a standard set of benefits for each American.

Emanuel, Ezekiel J. (2014). *Reinventing American Health Care: How the Affordable Care Act Will Improve Our Terribly Complex, Blatantly Unjust, Outrageously Expensive, Grossly Inefficient, Error Prone System.* New York: Public Affairs.

This book by a well-known scholar on medical ethics reviews the American healthcare system, healthcare reform efforts with a major focus on the ACA, and some thoughts on the future of healthcare and healthcare reform in the United States, including implementation problems with the ACA.

Field, Robert I. (2014). *Mother of Invention: How the Government Created Free-Market Health Care.* Oxford: Oxford University Press.

This book traces the government's role in building four key healthcare sectors into the financial powerhouses they are today: pharmaceuticals, hospitals, the medical profession, and private insurance. It traces their history, surveys their growth, and highlights some of their greatest success stories, which together reveal the indispensable role of public initiatives in contemporary private healthcare.

Gray, Virginia, Jennifer K. Benz, and David Lowery. (2013). *Interest Groups and Health Care Reform across the United States, 2013*. Washington, DC: Georgetown University Press.

The healthcare reform debate is complex, as the healthcare segment represents almost 20 percent of the U.S. economy and impacts the health and well-being of the entire population. Many groups representing the interests of political, economic, or demographic groups have been and are now very actively trying to influence the debate. This book focuses on interest representation and its involvement and impact on the health reform debate.

Institute of Medicine. (2001). *Crossing the Quality Chasm: A New Health System for the 21st Century*. Washington, DC: National Academy of Sciences.

This report argues that the nation's healthcare industry has foundered in its ability to provide safe, high-quality care consistently to all Americans and argues that reorganization and reform are needed to fix what is now a disjointed and inefficient system. One recommendation is that Congress create an "innovation fund" of $1 billion to help subsidize promising projects. The report also recommends that the U.S. Department of Health and Human Services monitor and track quality improvements in six key areas: safety, effectiveness, responsiveness to patients, timeliness, efficiency, and equity.

Institute of Medicine. (1999). *To Err Is Human*. Washington, DC: National Academy of Sciences.

This report from the Institute of Medicine found that more people die in the United States from medical mistakes each year than from highway accidents, breast cancer, or AIDS. One reason for this is that America's health system is a tangled, highly fragmented web that often wastes resources by providing unnecessary services and duplicating efforts, leaving unaccountable gaps in care and failing to build on the strengths of all health professionals.

Jacobs, Larry, and Theda Skopcol. (2012). *Health Care Reform and American Politics: What Everyone Needs to Know,* rev. and updated ed. New York: Oxford University Press.

In this updated edition, two of the nation's leading experts on politics and healthcare policy provide a concise and accessible overview. They explain the political battles of 2009 and 2010, highlighting White House strategies, the deals Democrats cut with interest groups, and the impact of agitation by Tea Partiers and progressives. Jacobs and Skopcol spell out what the new law can do for everyday Americans, what it will cost, and who will pay. In a new section, they also analyze the impact of the U.S. Supreme Court ruling that upheld the law. Above all, they explain what comes next, as critical yet often behind-the-scenes battles rage over implementing reform at the federal level and in the 50 states. Affordable care still faces challenges at the state level despite the court ruling. But, like Social Security and Medicare, it could also gain strength and popularity as the majority of Americans learn what it can do for them.

Jonas, Steven, Raymond L. Goldsteen, Karen Goldsteen, and S. Jonas. (2013). *Jonas' Introduction to the U.S. Health Care System,* 7th ed. New York: Springer.

The seventh and newest edition of this long-running textbook provides a balanced and concise introduction to the U.S. healthcare system. The new edition includes recent developments such as the significance of the rise of the Tea Party in the healthcare reform debate as well as passage of the act.

Kominski, Gerald F. (Ed.). (2014). *Changing the U.S. Health Care System: Key Issues in Health Services Policy and Management*, 4th ed. San Francisco: Jossey-Bass.

The fourth edition of this book presents essays from experts on a wide range of topics relating to healthcare management and policy.

Kotlikoff, Laurence J. (2007). *The Healthcare Fix: Universal Insurance for all Americans*. Cambridge, MA: Massachusetts Institute of Technology Press.

This book argues that both Medicare and Medicaid at their current rates of growth represent a threat to the nation's finances. The author proposes a Medical Security System (MSS) as a plan for single-payer universal health insurance that he believes would help solve the healthcare crisis and the health finance crisis. The system would involve universal vouchers that would be used to purchase health insurance, and thus, although the author uses the term "single payer," his approach is quite different from what most authors mean by a single-payer model for healthcare reform.

Kronenfeld, Jennie Jacobs. (2011). *Medicare/Health Care*. Westport, CT: Greenwood/ABC-CLIO.

This book reviews Medicare's history, explores its current coverages, and takes a look at its future. This includes issues such as drug coverage, HMO options, the lack of most long-term care coverage, and the demographic-based funding crisis.

Kronenfeld, Jennie Jacobs. (2006). *Expansion of Publicly Funded Health Insurance in the United States: The Children's Health Insurance Program and Its Implications*. Lanham, MD: Lexington Books.

This book focuses on issues of publicly funded health insurance in the United States, beginning with a review of Medicare and Medicaid. Much of the rest of the book focuses on the SCHIP program, special issues of children's access to healthcare services, and a case study of Arizona and attempts to improve enrollment rates both in Medicaid and in the new SCHIP program in Arizona (known as KidsCare).

Lister, John. (2013). *Health Policy Reform: Global Health versus Private Profit.* Faringdon, England: Libri.
    This book presents key issues facing health professionals today and explores the barrage of policies that threaten to deny them the right to deliver quality healthcare. The book's use of a common analytical framework produces a consistent critical analysis of different situations in various countries, making its approach wholly unlike previous studies of the topic of modern healthcare.

McDonough, John E., and Fund Milbank Memorial. (2011). *Inside National Health Reform.* Berkeley: University of California Press.
    This book provides an insider's view of the legislative efforts to reform the U.S. healthcare system that resulted in passage of the Affordable Care Act. It shows the large numbers of issues addressed and interest groups actively engaged in the effort. It covers the time period from President Obama's election in 2008 until passage of the law in 2010.

Quadagno, Jill. (2005). *One Nation Uninsured: Why the U.S. Has No National Health Insurance.* New York: Oxford University Press.
    This book by a medical sociologist reviews issues in the organization of healthcare in the United States across the twentieth century. Quadagno shows that each attempt to enact national health insurance was attacked by powerful stakeholders within healthcare. These groups often mobilized to keep the financing of healthcare away from the

government, especially prior to the passage of Medicare and Medicaid. After that, Quadagno argues the insurance industry assumed a leading role against reform.

Skopcol, Theda. (1992). *Protecting Soldiers and Mothers: The Political Origins of Social Policy in the United States.* Cambridge, MA: Harvard University Press.

Skocpol is a well-known sociologist who has brought historical, institutional, and comparative approaches to the study of the role of the state in much of her work. In this book, she conducts a historical analysis of the American welfare state, with a focus on programs linked to deserving groups in society, such as soldiers, their dependents, and mothers and their children.

Starr, Paul. (2013). *Remedy and Reaction: The Peculiar American Struggle over Health Care Reform, Revised Edition.* New Haven, CT: Yale University Press.

This book reviews the historical development of the U.S. healthcare system. The author's thesis is that this system has not developed in the same way as systems in other developed countries because of a history of satisfying the needs of enough of the public while allowing the development of an entrenched healthcare industry that greatly profits from the system has made reform extremely difficult.

Starr, Paul. (1984). *Social Transformation of American Medicine.* New York: Basic Books.

Winner of the 1983 Pulitzer Prize and the Bancroft Prize in American History, this is a landmark history of how the entire American healthcare system of doctors, hospitals, health plans, and government programs has evolved over the past two centuries.

Stevens, Rosemary. (1989). *In Sickness and in Wealth: American Hospitals in the Twentieth Century.* New York: Basic Books.

This book focuses on American hospitals, beginning with historical material from the beginning of the twentieth century and moving through the date of publication. The book explains how American hospitals became one of the central healthcare institutions by the 1960s and 1970s.

Journal Articles

Antos, Joseph R, Mark V. Pauly, and Gail R. Wilensky. (2012, September 6). Bending the Cost Curve through Market-Based Incentives. *New England Journal of Medicine* 367(10): 956. DOI: 10.1056/NEJMsb1207996.
   This article presents a conservative market approach to controlling healthcare costs.

Berkowitz, S. A., G. Gerstenblith, and G. F. Anderson. (2007). Medicare Prescription Drug Coverage Gap. *JAMA* 297(8): 868–870.
   This is a commentary on the problems with the Medicare prescription coverage gap often referred to as the donut hole.

Brennan, Troyen A., and David M. Studdert. (2010). How Will Health Insurers Respond to New Rules under Health Reform? *Health Affairs* 29(6): 1147–1151.
   The Obama health reform legislation creates many new rules for all groups involved in healthcare, especially for health insurers. This article reviews the statutes that are part of the new law and speculates on what the new regulations may be and the impact these will have on the health insurance industry. The authors argue the impact will especially change the small group and individual health insurance markets.

Brill, Steven. (2013, March 4). Bitter Pill: Why Medical Bills Are Killing Us. *Time.* healthland.time.com/2013/02/20/bitter-pill-why-medical-bills-are-killing-us/print/ (Aug 2014).

This story in *Time* magazine looks at why medical bills are so high and reviews the challenges in spending over 20 percent of the United States' GDP on healthcare.

Brooks, Tricia. (2014, June). Open Enrollment, Take Two. *Health Affairs* 33:927–930.
Even with the large problems in the launch of the enrollment process through the new health insurance marketplaces in 2013, the final enrollment figures were larger than projected. This article reviews how the enrollment process can be improved for the next open enrollment period.

Chernew, Michael, Davic M. Cutler, and Patricia Seliger Keenan. (2005, August). Increasing Health Insurance Costs and the Decline in Health Insurance Coverage. *Health Services Research* 40(4): 1021–1039.
This analysis was based on two cohorts of nonelderly Americans residing in 64 large metropolitan statistical areas (MSAs) surveyed in the Current Population Survey in 1989–1991 and 1998–2000. It found that the largest factor in the increase in the number of uninsured is the increase in the cost of this coverage.

Cohn Jonathan. (2010, May). How They Did It: An Inside Account of Health Care Reform's Triumph. *New Republic* 241(9): 14–25. http://www.newrepublic.com/article/75077/how-they-did-it.
As the title indicates, this story reviews how the administration and Democratic leaders were able to pass the Affordable Care Act.

Colla, Carrie H., Valeria A. Lewis, Stephen M. Shortell, and Elliott S. Fisher. (2014, June). First National Survey of ACOs Finds That Physicians Are Playing Strong Leadership and Ownership Roles. *Health Affairs*, 964–971.

This paper presents the findings of a national survey of accountable care organizations (ACOs) in 2012 and 2013. The authors found that physicians led or served on the boards of about 85 percent of ACOs. This level of physician leadership has important implications for the future evolution of ACOs. The authors indicate that the challenge of fundamentally changing care delivery as the country moves away from a fee-for-service structure will not be accomplished without strong, effective leadership from physicians.

Corrigan, Janet and McNeill, Dwight. (2009). Building Organizational Capacity: A Cornerstone of Health Care Reform. *Health Affairs* 28(2): w205–w215.

This article states that one requirement for successful reform of the U.S. healthcare system is the development of greater organizational capacity, including information technology. It calls for a comprehensive policy agenda to encourage this growth in organizational capacity, including national priorities and goals, performance measurement and reporting, payment reform, community leadership, information technology (IT), and public education.

Crosson, Francis J. (2009). Medicare: The Place to Start Delivery System Reform. *Health Affairs* 28(2): w232–234.

Crosson argues that the Medicare program should be used for developing accountable care organizations (ACOs) to develop transformations in payment design, incentives, and delivery system structure.

Cutler, David. (2010). Analysis and Commentary: How Health Care Reform Must Bend the Cost Curve. *Health Affairs* 29(6): 1131–1135.

This article argues that the true measure of healthcare reform's success will be whether it results in lowered medical costs over the long term. Features within the act that are designed to modernize the delivery of services and lead to a more efficient and effective healthcare system are discussed. These include bundling medical services into larger payment groups, value-based purchasing, and improvement of care coordination.

Dranove, David, Crag Garthwaite, and Christopher Ody. (2014, August). Health Spending Slowdown Is Mostly Due to Economic Factors, Not Structural Change in the Health Care Sector. *Health Affairs* 33:1399–1406.

The authors use data to support their thesis that the slowdown in the increase in healthcare costs was caused more by the downturn of the economy than by basic structural changes in the healthcare sector.

Emmanuel, Ezekial, Neera Tanden, Stuart Altman, Scott Armstrong, Donald Berwick, Maura Caslyn, et al. (2012, September). A Systematic Approach to Containing Health Care Spending. *New England Journal of Medicine* 367: 949–954. DOI: 10.1056/NEJMsb1205901.

This article reviews alternate strategies to control healthcare spending in the United States.

Guterman, S., Karen Davis, Kristof Stremikis, and Heather Drake. (2010). Innovation in Medicare and Medicaid Will Be Central to Health Reform's Success. *Health Affairs* 29(6): 1188–1193.

This article discusses aspects of the recent health reform legislation signed by Obama. The focus is on the innovations included for Medicare and Medicaid, especially those related to payment reform provisions. The article presents recommendations that the authors believe would maximize the effectiveness of a new center to deal with these reforms, which it argues are central to the success of health reform.

Hacker, Jacob, and Theodore Marmor. (2003). Medicare Reform: Fact, Fiction and Foolishness. *Public Policy and Aging Report* 13(4): 1–23.

> This article reviews the politics of Medicare after the major revisions in 2003. It focuses on the politics of crisis that drive the debate.

Halpin, Helen A., and Peter Harbage. (2010). The Origins and Demise of the Public Option. *Health Affairs* 29(6): 1117–1124.

> This article discusses the background of the public option for health insurance, the debate over whether this approach should be included as part of Obama's health-care reforms, and how it ended up being omitted from the final package adopted by both houses of Congress in March 2010.

Holtz-Eakin, Douglas, and Michael J. Ramlet. (2010). Health Care Reform Is Likely to Widen Federal Budget Deficits, Not Reduce Them. *Health Affairs* 29(6): 1136–1141.

> This article deals with the federal government's fiscal outlook and how the Patient Protection and Affordable Health Care Act is likely to impact it in coming years. Although the official Congressional Budget Office analysis suggested modest deficit reduction over the next decade, these authors argue that those conclusions are questionable and are based on omitted costs, premiums shifted from other entitlements, and the assumption of certain spending cuts and revenue increases.

Kahn, Charles N., III. (2009). Payment Reform Alone Will Not Transform Health Care Delivery. *Health Affairs* 28(2): w216–w218.

> While payment reforms are an important part of health reform, Kahn states that to maximize the chances of success and minimize the possibility of unintended consequences, the appropriate culture and structure of our healthcare institutions first must be in place.

Kingsdale, Jon, and John Bertko. (2010). Insurance Exchanges under Health Reform: Six Design Issues for the States. *Health Affairs* 29(6): 1158–1163.

This article discusses issues linked to the formation of health exchanges as part of Obama's health reforms and points out that many important issues are not resolved by the legislation; rather, they are left to the states. To successfully implement the legislation, private-public partnerships will be needed. States will need more expertise in insurance operations and marketing.

Laugesen, Miriam J. (2009). Siren Song: Physicians, Congress and Medicare Fees. *Journal of Health Politics, Policy and Law* 34(2): 157–179.

Physician fees are adjusted annually based on a formula called the sustainable growth rate (SGR). Physician groups have successfully fought in Congress changes that would reduce fees while supporting changes that increase fees. Policymakers need to resist physician groups, balancing lobbying pressure with broader cost-containment goals.

Miller, Thomas P. (2010). Health Reform: Only a Cease-Fire in a Political Hundred Years War. *Health Affairs* 29(6): 1101–1105.

This article views four major political forces as having been important in the reform debates of the past two years: federal budget constraints, public concerns about the size and reach of the federal government, time pressure of the congressional calendar, and issues surrounding the political parties and the Obama administration. The article argues that passage of the legislation is a success at this point but really more of a "cease-fire" in a long-standing debate between forces for implementation and forces for repeal and replace.

Oberlander, Jonathan. (2012, August 16). Unfinished Journey: A Century of Health Care Reform. *New England Journal of Medicine* 367(7): 585–590.

> This Perspectives piece reviews the federal government's efforts to develop and reform the healthcare system. It includes a time line of these efforts.

Oberlander, Jonathan. (2010). Long Time Coming: Why Health Care Reform Finally Passed. *Health Affairs* 29(6): 1112–1116.

> This article discusses why the Obama administration was able to win some health reforms in 2009–2010, in contrast to failed earlier efforts. They argue that the Democrats and the Obama administration learned from past failures, and they especially emphasize the importance of neutralizing interest groups.

Quadagno, Jill. (2014, February). Right Wing Conspiracy? Socialist Plot? The Origins of the Patient Protection and Affordable Care Act. *Journal of Health Politics, Policy and Law* 39: 35–56.

> This article shows that the Affordable Care Act was neither a first step to socialism as claimed by conservative critics or a sellout as claimed by left-leaning critics wanting a true single-payer system. The author shows how it has elements of both views and a legacy of the Clinton health reform initiatives from 10 years earlier.

Smyrl, Marc E. (2014, February). Beyond Interests and Institutions: US Health Policy Reform and the Surprising Silence of Big Business. *Journal of Health Politics, Policy and Law* 39: 5–34.

> In the healthcare reform debate leading to the passing of the Affordable Care Act, many major U.S. employers did not take an active role in the debate. The authors analyze why, identifying the conflicting principles of corporate

self-interest and the corporate provision of "welfare" services such as healthcare and retirement.

Sorenson, Corinna, Michael K Gusmano, and Adam Oliver. (2014, February). The Politics of Comparative Effectiveness Research: Lessons from Recent History. *Journal of Health Politics, Policy and Law* 39: 139–170.
> This article reviews previous initiatives in the use of comparative effectiveness research to identify the most effective medical treatments. The article highlights their prescribed role in U.S. healthcare, the reasons for their success or failure, and the political lessons learned. It also discusses how current CER initiatives have corrected for many of the pitfalls experienced by previous efforts.

Steinmo, Sven and Jon Watts. (1995). It's the Institutions, Stupid! Why Comprehensive National Health Insurance Always Fails in America. *Journal of Health Politics, Policy and Law* 20 (2): 329–372.
> This article argues that the United States does not have comprehensive national health insurance because American political institutions are biased against this type of reform. It discusses the fragmented American polity and how this has led to fragmented efforts at reform of the health system.

Weinstein, Milton C. (2001). Should Physicians Be Gatekeepers of Medical Resources? *Journal of Medical Ethics* 27: 268–274.
> This article argues that the physician's responsibilities to provide the best available medical care conflict with our country's need to best spend our available resources and that physicians thus cannot serve as the gatekeeper for access to these services.

Reports

As discussed in earlier chapters, the healthcare industry represents more than 15 percent of the U.S. economy and is vital to all citizens. Therefore, there are many nonprofit issue advocacy groups representing the various players such as physicians, consumers, government policymakers, insurance companies, and so forth. The sites discussed in this section contain news, analysis, and data relating to the healthcare system and to health reform, but be sure to look at who the groups represent and if they come from a specific political viewpoint. The next section presents information on sites that provide access to relevant reports relating to healthcare reform.

The Alliance for Health Reform (http://www.allhealth.org/) is a major nonpartism coalition studying health reform and how to provide health coverage for all Americans at a reasonable cost. Democratic senator Jay Rockefeller of West Virginia and Republican senator Roy Blunt of Missouri serve as honorary chairs of the coalition. The alliance produces toolkits, issue briefs, and reports on major topics related to healthcare, including health reform. With funding from the Robert Wood Johnson Foundation, they publish a concise review of significant health topics for reporters.

The Alliance for Health Reform. *Covering Health Issues: A Source Book for Reporters* (http://www.allhealth.org/source bookTOC.asp?SBID=7) provides a concise but detailed presentation on the topics covered.

American Health Insurance Plans (AHIP) (http://www.ahip .org/) is the professional organization representing health insurance providers. In representing the health insurance industry, it has lobbied again key aspects of the Democratic health reform legislation passed in March 2010 that significantly impact their industry. The following reports are useful in researching health reform.

American Health Insurance Plans (AHIP). (2013, November). *A Roadmap to High Quality Affordable Health Care for All Americans.* (http://www.americanhealthsolution.org/ Workarea/DownloadAsset.aspx?id=214749503).

This report reviews current research listing key drivers of healthcare costs and advances a new policy framework for bending the cost curve and improving the quality of patient care.

Milliman, Inc. for American Health Insurance Plans (AHIP). *Report: Comprehensive Assessment of ACA Factors That Will Affect Individual Market Premiums in 2014.* (http://www.americanhealthsolution.org/Workarea/Download Asset.aspx?id=2147491347). This report provides a comprehensive assessment and review of the major factors affecting national health insurance premiums in the ACA individual health market.

Cato Institute (www.cato.org/) is a nonprofit libertarian think tank located in Washington, DC, "dedicated to the principles of individual liberty, limited government, free markets and peace." It is nonpartisan in its support of smaller government and less government involvement and regulation in all aspects of American society. Cato publishes a large number of reports and books supporting its positions. It strongly opposed President Obama's health reform programs in the 2009–2010 debates. Its Health Care and Welfare section (http://www. cato.org/research/health-care) presented the following report published in January 2014 relating to ACA from the libertarian perspective:

Tanner, Michael. (2014, January 27). *Policy Analysis 745, Obama Care: What We Know Now.* (http://object.cato .org/sites/cato.org/files/pubs/pdf/pa745_web_1.pdf).

Center for American Progress (CAP) (http://www.american progress.org) is a progressive think tank strongly supportive of health reform to move the United States toward universal healthcare. CAP was founded in 2003 by John Podesta, who served as White House chief of staff in the Clinton administration. CAP lobbies for liberal, progressive solutions in

a wide area of national and international issues (http://www
.americanprogress.org/about/our-issues/). Its website's health reform (http://www.americanprogress.org/issues/healthcare/view/)
page links to a number of reports such as:

> Emanuel Ezekiel, Topher Spiro, Maura Calsyn, Carter
> Price, Stuart Altman, Scott Armstrong, et al. (2014,
> August). *Accountable Care States: The Future of Health
> Care Cost Control.* (http://cdn.americanprogress.org/wp
> -content/uploads/2014/09/AccountableCareStates.pdf).

> Tanden, Neera, Zeke Emanuel, and Topher Spiro. (2014,
> May 17). *A New Management Structure for a New Phase of
> the Affordable Care Act.* (http://cdn.americanprogress.org/
> wp-content/uploads/2014/05/ACAmngment_0517.pdf)

> Tanden, Neera, Zeke Emanuel, Topher Spiro, Emily
> Oshima Lee, and Thomas Huelskoetter. (2014, January
> 24). *Comparing the Effectiveness of Health Care Fulfilling
> the Mission of the Patient-Centered Outcomes Research Ins-
> titute.* (http://cdn.americanprogress.org/wp-content/uploads/
> 2014/01/ComparativeEffectiveness2.pdf)

> Spiro, Topher, and Jonathan Gruber. (2013, October
> 21). *The Affordable Care Act's Lower-Than-Projected
> Premiums Will Save $190 Billion.* (http://cdn.american
> progress.org/wp-content/uploads/2013/10/SpiroACASavings
> -brief.pdf)

Center for Children and Families (CCF) (http://ccf.george
town.edu/) is an independent, nonpartisan policy and research
center working to expand and improve health coverage for
America's children and families. Based at Georgetown University's Health Policy Institute, CCF works to accomplish this
by finding ways to improve access to, and the quality of,
healthcare for children and families, especially for the poor
and working class. Its website provides updated information
on the Affordable Care Act, Medicaid, and Children's Health

Insurance Program (CHIP). Below are three of the reports related to health reform and children.

Brooks, Tricia, and Martha Heberlein. (2014, April). *Renewing Medicaid and CHIP under the Affordable Care Act.* (http://ccf.georgetown.edu/wp-content/uploads/2014/04/Renewing-Medicaid-and-CHIP-Under-the-ACA.pdf)

Kenney, Genevieve M., Joan Alker, Nathaniel Anderson, Stacey McMorrow, Sharon K. Long, Douglas Wissoker, et al. (2014, September).*A First Look at Uninsured Rate for Children since Major Affordable Care Act Provisions Took Effect.* (http://ccf.georgetown.edu/wp-content/uploads/2014/09/A-First-Look-at-Childrens-Health-Insurance-Coverage-under-the-ACA-in-2014-wlogo.pdf). This report was jointly prepared by CCF and Urban Institute researchers and is listed on the CCF website.

Medicaid Provides Needed Access to Care. (2014, April). (http://ccf.georgetown.edu/wp-content/uploads/2013/11/access-factsheet.pdf)

The Commonwealth Fund (http://www.cmwf.org) describes itself as a "private foundation that aims to promote a high performing health care system that achieves better access, improved quality, and greater efficiency, particularly for society's most vulnerable, including low-income people, the uninsured, minority Americans, young children, and elderly adults." (http://www.commonwealthfund.org/About-Us.aspx) The site provides extensive information on the following topics:

- Health system performance
- Healthcare delivery
- Health coverage
- Patient-centered care
- Vulnerable populations
- Medicare

- State health policy
- Affordable Care Act reforms
- International health policy
- Payment reform

Examples of recent Commonwealth Fund Reports relevant to health reform include:

Schoen, Cathy, Susan L. Hayes, Sara R. Collins, Jacob A. Lippa, and David C. Radley. (2014, March). *America's Underinsured: A State-by-State Look at Health Insurance Affordability Prior to the New Coverage Expansions* (http://www.commonwealthfund.org/publications/fund -reports/2014/mar/americas-underinsured#).

Collins, Sara R. (2014, February). *Young Adult Participation in the Health Insurance Marketplaces: Just How Important Is It?* (http://www.commonwealthfund .org/~/media/files/publications/fund-report/2014/feb/1732 _collins_young_adult_participation_hlt_ins_marketplaces _v2.pdf).

Keith, Katie, and Kevin W. Lucia. (2014, January). *Implementing the Affordable Care Act: The State of the States.* (http://www.commonwealthfund.org/~/media/files/ publications/fund-report/2014/jan/1727_keith_implementing _aca_state_of_states.pdf).

Schoen, Cathy, David Radley, Pamela Riley, Jacob Lippa, Julia Berenson, Cara Dermody, and Anthony Shih. (2013, September). *Health Care in the Two Americas: Findings from the Scorecard on State Health System Performance for Low-Income Populations, 2013.* (http://www.commonwealthfund .org/~/media/files/publications/fund-report/2013/sep/1700 _schoen_low_income_scorecard_full_report_final_v4.pdf).

Families USA (http://www.familiesusa.org) is an advocacy group that describes itself as "a national nonprofit, non-partisan organization dedicated to the achievement of high-quality, afford-able health and long-term care for all Americans." It strongly supported passage of the Affordable Care Act and is trying to assist people eligible for healthcare coverage via ACA to enroll. The following report focuses on steps to increase enrollment at the next open enrollment period

Pollack, Ron, and Rachel Klein. (2014, April). *Accelerating the Affordable Care Act's Enrollment Momentum: 10 Recommendations for Future Enrollment Periods.* (http://familiesusa.org/sites/default/files/product _documents/ENR_Enrollment_report_FINAL_032814_web .pdf).

The Galen Institute (http://www.galen.org/) is a nonprofit, Section 501(c)(3) public policy research organization sup-porting a free market approach to healthcare to create a patient-centered health sector. They publish numerous reports and commentaries representing their view, including:

Turner, Grace-Marie. (2014, Summer). How to Get a Health Care System That Answers to the Patient. *Insider*, pp. 22–31. (http://www.insideronline.org/archives/2014/ summer/HealthCare.pdf).

HCCI Health Care Cost Institute (http://www.health costinstitute.org), founded in 2011, states that its mission is to promote independent research and analysis on the causes of rising U.S. health spending, to provide policymakers, con-sumers, and researchers with better, more transparent infor-mation on what is driving healthcare costs and to help ensure that, over time, the nation is able to get greater value from its health spending. Through its website, it presents its semiannual report on healthcare costs.

2012 Health Care Cost and Utilization Report (2013, September). (http://www.healthcostinstitute.org/2012report).

Health Research Institute (HRI) (http://www.pwc.com/us/ en/health-industries/health-research-institute/index.jhtml) is a component of PWC (PricewaterhouseCoopers), which is a top 500 company and the world's second-largest professional services network. HRI provides information on, perspectives on, and analysis of trends affecting health-related industries. The following report presents its projection for the coming year's medical cost trend based on activity in the market that serves employer-based insurance:

> *Medical Cost Trends: Behind the Numbers.* (2014, June). (http://www.pwc.com/us/en/health-industries/behind-the-numbers/index.jhtml)

The Henry J. Kaiser Family Foundation (http://www.kff.org/) is a California-based foundation that is an independent nonprofit national healthcare philanthropy that focuses on a variety of healthcare and health policy concerns. Its focus is providing up-to-date information on major health issues through Kaiser Foundation research and bring together research and information from other sources in a clearinghouse-type function. Recent reports accessible via its website include:

> Hamel, Liz, Mira Rao, Larry Levitt, Gary Claxton, Cynthia Cox, Karen Pollitz, and Mollyann Brodie. *Survey of Non-Group Health Insurance Enrollees.* (http://kff.org/private-insurance/report/survey-of-non-group-health-insurance-enrollees/).

> Pollitz, Karen, Cynthia Cox, Kevin Lucia, and Katie Keith. (2014, January). *Medical Debt among People with Health Insurance.* (http://kaiserfamilyfoundation.files.wordpress.com/2014/01/8537-medical-debt-among-people-with-health-insurance.pdf).

The Heritage Foundation (http://www.heritage.org/) is a conservative think tank whose mission is to "formulate and promote conservative public policies based on the principles of free enterprise, limited government, individual freedom, traditional American values, and a strong national defense." Its Health Care page (http://www.heritage.org/issues/health-care)

provides access to Heritage-sponsored reports and blog updates on the healthcare system and health reform from a conservative viewpoint. Several recent reports relevant to healthcare reform are:

Moffit, Robert E., and Alyene Senger. (2014, September). *Progress in Medicare Advantage: Key Lessons for Medicare Reform.* (http://thf_media.s3.amazonaws.com/2014/pdf/B G2945.pdf).

Pope, Christopher M. (2014, August). *How the Affordable Care Act Fuels Health Care Market Consolidation.* (http:// thf_media.s3.amazonaws.com/2014/pdf/BG2928.pdf).

Haislmaier, Edmund F., and Drew Gonshorowski. (2014, July 28). *New Obamacare Enrollment Data: Employer-Based Coverage Declines.* (http://thf_media.s3.amazonaws .com/2014/pdf/BG2933.pdf).

National Academy for State Health Policy (NASHP) (http:// www.nashp.org) is a nonprofit, nonpartisan organization set up to analyze health reform and policy on the state level. NASHP works with individual states to deal with key health-related issues such as coverage and access, chronic and long-term care, health system improvement, and specific populations. It provides access reports on specific issues on the state level effort on implementation of health reform. Three of these reports are:

Wirth, Barbara, Charles Townley, and Mary Takach. (2014, August). *A Roadmap for State Policymakers to Use Comparative Effectiveness and Patient-Centered Outcomes Research to Inform Decision Making.* (http://www.nashp .org/sites/default/files/Roadmap.final_.8.6.2014.pdf).

Snyder, Andrew, Keerti Kanchinadam, Catherine Hess, and Rachel Dolan. (2014, April). *Improving Integration of Dental Health Benefits in Health Insurance Marketplaces.* (http://www.nashp.org/sites/default/files/improving.integration

.of_.dental.health.benefits.in_.health.insurance.market
places_0.pdf, Sept 20145).

Stanek, Michael. (2014, February). *Quality Measurement
to Support Value-Based Purchasing: Aligning Federal and
State Efforts.* (http://www.nashp.org/sites/default/files/
Quality.Measurement.Support.ValueBasedPurchasing.pdf).

National Center for Policy Analysis (http://www.ncpa.org) is
a private policy-oriented group that publishes material on a variety of policy topics, including healthcare policy. It has a more
conservative point of view and lists its mission as "Developing
and providing private alternatives to government regulation" in
a variety of public policy areas. The group covers health, Social
Security, welfare, criminal justice, environmental, and educational issues. Many of the reports are more in-depth examinations
of topics, rather than responses to a specific new proposal.
NCPA's healthcare page (http://www.ncpa.org/healthcare/) is
Free-Market Health Care Policy: Unique, One-of-a-Kind
Solutions, reflecting the group's conservative approach. It links
to information on health policy and reform topics presenting
the conservative perspective. Several of its reports relevant to
health reform are:

Goodwin, J. C. (2001, April). *Characteristics of an Ideal
Health Care System,* Policy Report 242 (http://www
.ncpa.org/pdfs/st242.pdf).

Herrick, Devon M. (2014, June). *The Effects of the
Affordable Care Act on Small Business,* Policy Report 356
(http://www.ncpa.org/pdfs/st356.pdf).

Graham, John R. T. (2014, May 29). *The Biggest Myths of
ObamaCare,* Issue Brief 144. (http://www.ncpa.org/pdfs/
ib144.pdf).

The National Coalition on Healthcare (http://www.nchc
.org/) is nonprofit and self-proclaimed rigorously nonpartisan

coalition of almost 80 groups employing or representing approximately 50 million Americans. A listing of its membership is available on its website. Its focus is examining health-related issues to look at ways to achieve better, more affordable healthcare for all Americans. The coalition represents more than 80 participating organizations, including medical societies, businesses, unions, healthcare providers, faith-based associations, pension and health funds, insurers, and groups representing consumers, patients, women, minorities, and persons with disabilities. The coalition focuses on effective healthcare reform while controlling the cost of healthcare. Its public education efforts focus on increasing understanding of the impact of health cost and quality problems on our nation's physical and financial health. Its policy page (http://www.nchc.org/policy/) presents its plan for improving healthcare while controlling cost, relevant fact sheets, issue briefs, and its report on U.S. healthcare growth.

Curbing Costs, Improving Care: The Path to an Affordable Health Care Future. (2010). (http://www.nchcbeta.org/wp-content/uploads/2012/05/NCHC-Plan-for-Health-and-Fiscal-Policy.pdf).

Mcneely, Larry. (2013). *Curbing Health Costs, Improving Quality: Care for High Cost Beneficiaries in Medicare and Medicaid.* (http://nchcbeta.org/wp-content/uploads/2013/05/Policy-Brief-High-Cost-Beneficiaries.pdf).

Mcneely, Larry. (2013). *Curbing Health Costs, Improving Quality: Towards New Models of Provider Payment.* (http://nchcbeta.org/wp-content/uploads/2013/05/Policy-Brief-Provider-Payment.pdf).

National Health Policy Forum (NHPF) (http://www.nhpf.org) is located at George Washington University in Washington, DC, and provides a forum for a nonpartisan exchange of ideas between senior government staff and experts from many healthcare setting. The site provides summaries of these sessions and to the reports that came out of many of them, two of which are:

Cunningham, Rob. (2013, October). *Health Workforce Needs: Projections Complicated by Practice and Technology Changes.* (http://www.nhpf.org/library/issue-briefs/IB851 _WorkforceProjections_10-22-13.pdf).

Linehan, Kathryn. (2013, July 19). *Medicare Advantage Update: Benefits, Enrollment, and Payments after the ACA.* (http://www.nhpf.org/library/issue-briefs/IB850_MAUpdate _07-19-13.pdf).

National Institute for Health Care Reform (http://www .nihcr.org/) is a 501(c)(3) nonprofit, nonpartisan organization established by the International Union, UAW; Chrysler Group LLC; Ford Motor Company; and General Motors to conduct health policy research and analysis to improve the organization, financing, and delivery of healthcare in the United States. Its publications page (http://www.nihcr.org/Publications) provides brief descriptions with links to the full publication for issue briefs and articles published in health policy journals on health policy and health reform, two of which are:

Grossman, Joy M., Rebecca Gourevitch, and Dori Cross. (2014, July). *Hospital Experiences Using Electronic Health Records to Support Medication Reconciliation.* (http://www .nihcr.org/index.php?download=1tlcfl362).

Abraham, Jean M., Peter Graven, and Roger Feldman. (2012, December). *Employer-Sponsored Insurance and Health Reform: Doing the Math,* Research Brief 11. (http://www.nihcr.org/index.php?download=1tlcfl201).

Physicians for a National Health Program (http://www .pnhp.org/) is an association of physicians who advocate a single-payer national healthcare system. This group does both issue analysis and advocacy, and it provides a liberal analysis of how to deal with healthcare reform, given its advocacy of a single-payer system. Its website provides links to the latest news, research, proposals, single-payer resources, getting active, multimedia and slide shows. In 2003, the group published a special commentary in *JAMA* with its proposal for a national healthcare system that is still relevant:

> Physician's Working Group for Single-Payer National Health Insurance. (2003, august 13). Proposal of the Physicians' Working Group for Single-Payer National Health Insurance. *JAMA*, 90(6): 797–805. (http://www.pnhp.org/PDF_files/Physicians%20ProposalJAMA.pdf).

Rand (http://www.rand.org/) is a major public policy oriented research institute that began during World War II and since then has become an independent nonprofit research and policy organization. With a staff of 1,700, of whom about 1,000 are research staff, Rand conducts research on a wide variety of public policy topics, including healthcare, education, and welfare. Rand's 2013 funding of over $63 million came from a number of sources, the largest of which is state, local and national government grants and projects. Rand also operates the Pardee Rand Graduate School, which, with about 100 PhD students, is the world's leading producer of doctorate-level public policy analysts. Health and healthcare is a focus area of Rand's research. The health and healthcare area page (http://www.rand.org/topics/health-and-health-care.html) provides links to numerous full-text reports and briefs, including:

> Carman, Katherine Grace, and Christine Eibner. (2014). *Changes in Health Insurance Enrollment since 2013: Evidence from the RAND Health Reform Opinion Study.* (http://www.rand.org/content/dam/rand/pubs/research_reports/RR600/RR656/RAND_RR656.pdf).

> Saltzman, Evan, and Christine Eibner. (2014). *Evaluating the "Keep Your Health Plan Fix" Implications for the Affordable Care Act Compared to Legislative Alternatives.*

(http://www.rand.org/content/dam/rand/pubs/research
_reports/RR500/RR529/RAND_RR529.pdf).

Rural Assistance Center (RAC) (http://www.raconline.org/)
was started in 2002 at the University of North Dakota. It serves
as an "information portal" for rural communities and others
to help provide quality health and human services to rural
residents. Its funding comes from the federal Office of Rural
Health Policy (ORHP) and stems from the U.S. Department of
Health and Human Services' Rural Initiative. RAC works with
states' offices of rural health and workforce agencies. The
group's website include topic pages that provide access to
reports, organizations, websites, funding opportunities, news,
and events relating to health policy issues related to rural
communities from various resources, including:

> Potter Andy, Matt Nattinger, and Keith J. Mueller;
> RUPRI Center for Rural Health Policy Analysis. (2014,
> September). *Rural Implications of the Blueprints for State-
> Based Health Insurance Marketplaces*. (http://www.public
> -health.uiowa.edu/rupri/publications/policypapers/Blueprints
> %20for%20State-Based%20Marketplaces.pdf).

> National Association of Community Health Centers.
> (2014, March). *Access Is the Answer: Community Health
> Centers, Primary Care & the Future of American Health
> Care*. (http://www.nachc.com/client/PIBrief14.pdf).

> Kaiser Family Foundation. (2013, October). *Health
> Coverage and Care for American Indians and Alaska
> Natives*. (http://kaiserfamilyfoundation.files.wordpress
> .com/2013/10/8502-health-coverage-and-care-for-american
> -indians-and-alaska-natives.pdf).

The State Health Access Data Assistance Center (SHADAC)
(http://www.shadac.org/) is an online resource providing data
for health policy research and analysis, including resources

related to issues of health insurance coverage, data collection methods, and state health policy. It is a program of the Robert Wood Johnson Foundation and part of the Health Policy and Management Division of the School of Public Health at the University of Minnesota. A good example of the data reports it produces is:

> Fried, Brett. (2014, February). *Geographic Concentration of the Uninsured: County-Level Estimates of Uninsurance.* (http://www.shadac.org/files/shadac/publications/Final Report_CountiesUninsured_Feb2014.pdf).

Edit   View   History   Bookmarks   Window   Help   Health Insurance Marketplace: Enroll for 201

https://www.healthcare.gov/

7D firmware...nload v2.0   7D firmware update–1   CD Pro Scan... Equipment   IN

regon – Google Search   Health Insurance Marketplace: En...

althCare.gov

Individuals & Families

Get Answers

Keep or Change Your Plan

et Coverage

See plans & prices fo

Starting November 15, you can enroll in an affordable health

GET READY TO E

SEE PLANS & PRICES

You may still be able to get coverage for the rest of 2014. Learn more.

HAVE A 2014 PLAN? STAY C

This chapter presents a chronology of important events relevant to healthcare and healthcare reform in the United States. It begins with the first acts of the federal government relating to health in the United States and focuses more heavily on the twentieth century forward. Within that time frame, more emphasis is placed on the period since the passage of the Medicare and Medicaid legislation in 1965, which led to a much greater focus on issues relating to healthcare at a national level.

1798   The Merchant Marine Services Act of 1798 is passed.

Early 1800s   The Merchant Marine Hospitals are established in major seaports of the United States, as authorized by the 1798 legislation.

1800   Legislation authorizes federal officials to cooperate with state and local officials to enforce quarantine laws.

A screenshot of the HealthCare.gov website, where people can buy health insurance, shown in Portland, Oregon. Being uninsured in America will cost you more in 2015. In 2015, all taxpayers have to report to the Internal Revenue Service for the first time whether or not they had health insurance the previous year. Most will check a box. It's also when the IRS starts collecting fines from some uninsured people, and deciding if others qualify for exemptions. (AP Photo/Don Ryan)

1862   The Morrill Act grants federal lands to each state and allows profits from those lands to be used to support public institutions of higher education.

President Lincoln appoints a chemist, Charles M. Wetherill, to serve in the new Department of Agriculture. This is the beginning of the Bureau of Chemistry, which was a forerunner to the Food and Drug Administration.

1870   The Marine Hospitals Services Act of 1870 creates a national agency with a central headquarters to oversee merchant marine hospitals and staffing.

1878   The Federal Quarantine Act of 1878 and subsequent amendments give the Marine Hospital Service the authority to develop quarantine laws for ports that lack state or local regulation.

1882   The first general immigration law includes provisions to exclude immigrants for medical reasons. Federal inspectors and doctors have to be allowed on board ships to check for diseases as a way to enforce these laws.

1887   The federal government opens a one-room laboratory on Staten Island for research on diseases. This agency eventually becomes the National Institutes of Health.

1899   The Commission Corps Act of 1899 and amendments allow the hiring of physicians and other health personnel to provide public heath services.

1901   The U.S. Health Service Hygienic Laboratory is established.

1902   The Public Health and Marine Service Act of 1902 clarifies some federal health functions by renaming Marine Hospital Services as the Public Health and Marine Services.

The Biologics Control Act of 1902 provides the Public Health Service with the responsibility of licensing and regulating biologically derived health products.

1906   The Pure Food and Drug Act of 1906 (Wiley Act) allows the Bureau of Chemistry in the Department of Agriculture to prohibit shipment of impure foods and drugs across state lines. It creates the ability to regulate drug products, and later to create specialized categories of drugs such as controlled substances.

1912 President Theodore Roosevelt's first White House Conference urges creation of a children's bureau to combat exploitation of children. The conference deals with many aspects of the lives of children, including health-related concerns.

1917 The Vocational Educational Act of 1917 (Smith-Hughes Act) provides funds to establish early licensed practical nursing (LPN) programs.

1920 The Snyder Act of 1920 is the first federal legislation to deal with healthcare for Native Americans.

1921 The Maternity and Infancy Act of 1921 (Sheppard-Towner Act) provides grants to states to plan maternal and child health services. Although the law is allowed to lapse in 1929, it was very important because the mechanism of providing grants to states was new within the health area. This legislation served as a prototype for federal grants in aid to states in the area of health.

1924 The Veterans Act of 1924 codifies and extends the role of the federal government in the provision of healthcare services to veterans.

1930 The Ransdell Act of 1930 creates the National Institutes of Health from the Hygienic Laboratory and sets in place the growth of federally funded health research.

The Veterans' Administration is created as an independent U.S. government agency.

1932 The Committee on the Costs of Medical Care report is published and raises concerns about the costs of medical care and the number of people who are effectively denied access to healthcare services due to costs and limited incomes.

1935 The Social Security Act of 1935, including Title V, is passed. This landmark legislation provides for a system of old age pensions and other old age benefits.

1937   The Social Security Act is expanded to include benefits for spouses and widows.

The National Cancer Institute is created; it later becomes part of the National Institutes of Health.

1938   The Federal Food, Drug, and Cosmetic Act of 1938 and amendments regulate market entry of new drug, cosmetic, and therapeutic products for safety. It extends federal authority to ban new drugs from the market until they are approved by the Food and Drug Administration (FDA).

The Venereal Disease Control Act of 1938 (LaFollette-Bulwinkle Act) coordinates state efforts to combat syphilis and gonorrhea by providing grants in aid to the states to support investigation and control of venereal disease.

1939   The Reorganization Act of 1939 realigns many health-related functions in the federal government.

1941   The Nurse Training Act of 1941 provides schools of nursing with support to increase enrollments and improve physical facilities.

1944   The Public Health Service Act of 1944 is passed; it is a large, multipart piece of legislation that makes many changes in the role of the federal government in public health services.

1945   The McCarran-Fergurson Act of 1945 exempts the business of insurance from federal antitrust legislation (such as the Sherman Antitrust Act of 1890 and the Clayton Act of 1914). Instead, insurance is to be regulated by state law.

1946   The U.S. National Health Policy Hospital Survey and Construction Act of 1946 (HillBurton Amendments to PHS) provides grants to states in order to inventory and survey existing hospital and public healthcare facilities in each state and to plan for new ones.

The National Mental Health Act of 1946 (amendment to the PHS act) authorizes federal support for mental health research and treatment programs.

1948   The National Health Act of 1948 expands the capacity of NIH by making it the National Institutes of Health and creating a second categorical institute, the National Heart Institute.

1953   The Federal Security Administration is renamed and given department status as the Department of Health, Education, and Welfare.

1954   The Medical Facilities Survey and Construction Act of 1954 (amendments to the Hill-Burton Act of 1946) greatly expands the program's scope by authorizing grants for surveys and construction of diagnostic and treatment centers, including hospital outpatient departments, chronic disease hospitals, rehabilitation facilities, and nursing homes.

1956   The Health Amendments Act of 1956 modifies the basic PHS Act of 1944 by adding special projects dealing with problems of state mental hospitals. It also provides federal assistance for the education and training of health personnel.

The Dependents Medical Care Act of 1956 establishes the Civilian Health and Medical Program of the Uniformed Services (CHAMPUS) for the dependents of military personnel.

1958   The Food Additives Amendment of 1958 amends the Food, Drug, and Cosmetic Act of 1938 to require premarketing clearance from the FDA for new food additives.

1959   The Federal Employees Health Benefit Act of 1959 permits Blue Cross to negotiate a contract with the Civil Service Commission to provide health insurance coverage for federal employees.

1960   The Social Security Amendments of 1960 (Kerr-Mills Act) amends the Social Security Act to establish a program of medical assistance for the aged.

1961   The Community Health Services and Facilities Act of 1961, although passed as a separate statue, mostly amends the Hill-Burton Act of 1946 by increasing the amount of funds available for nursing home construction and by extending the research and demonstration grant program to other medical facilities.

1962   The Health Services Act for Agricultural Migratory Workers Act of 1962 (amendment to the PHS Act) establishes a program of federal grants for family clinics and other health services for migrant workers and their families.

The Drug Amendments of 1962 (Kefauver-Harris Amendments) modifies the Food, Drug, and Cosmetic Act of 1938 to significantly strengthen the provisions related to the regulation of therapeutic drugs.

1963   The Maternal and Child Health and Mental Retardation Planning Amendments to Title V of the Social Security Act (including those in 1965 and 1967) modify the basic Social Security Act to assist states and communities in preventing and combating developmental disabilities through expansion and improvement of the maternal and child and crippled children's programs. It also adds special project grants for maternity and infant care for low-income mothers and infants and special project grants for child dental services.

The Health Professions Education Assistance Act of 1963 amends the PHS Act to provide construction grants for facilities that train physicians, nurses, dentists, podiatrists, pharmacists, and public health personnel.

1964   The first Surgeon General's Report on Smoking and Health is released, marking the beginning of growing public recognition of the negative health effects of smoking.

1965   The Health Professions Educational Assistance Amendments of 1965 amend the 1963 act by providing basic improvement (institutional) grants, special improvement grants, and scholarship grants to schools of medicine, dentistry, osteopathy, optometry, and podiatry.

The Health Insurance for the Aged of 1965 (Title XVIII of the Social Security Act) and amendments establish Medicare, a program of national health insurance for older adults who are Social Security recipients. Part A provides basic protection against the costs of hospital and selected post-hospital services. Part B is a voluntary program financed by premium payments from enrollees with matching federal revenues. It provides supplemental medical insurance benefits.

Title XIX of the Social Security Act (Medicaid) creates grants to the states for Medical Assistance Programs of 1965. These amendments create a federal-state matching program with voluntary state participation to partially replace Kerr-Mills.

The Older Americans Act of 1965 establishes the Administration on Aging to administer programs for older adults through state agencies

1966   The Comprehensive Health Planning and Public Health Service Amendments of 1966 (Partnership for Health) provide for state and local planning for health services facilities through A and B agencies.

1967   The Mental Health Amendments of 1967 and Mental Retardation Amendments to the Mental Retardation Facilities and Community Mental Health Centers Construction Act of 1965 extend construction grants to community mental health centers to cover acquisition of existing buildings. It also extends the program of construction grants for university-affiliated and community-based facilities for people with developmental disabilities.

The Social Security Amendments of 1967 are the first of many modifications to the Medicare and Medicaid programs established first by the Social Security Amendments of 1965.

1970   The Comprehensive Drug Abuse and Prevention and Control Act of 1970 provides for special project grants for drug abuse and drug dependence treatment programs and programs related to drug education.

The Poison Prevention and Packaging Act of 1970 requires that most drugs be dispensed in containers designed to be difficult for children to open.

The Comprehensive Alcohol Abuse and Alcoholism Prevention, Treatment, and Rehabilitation Act of 1970 establishes the National Institute of Alcohol Abuse and Alcoholism. The act also provides a separate statutory base for programs and activities relating to alcohol abuse and alcoholism.

The Communicable Disease Control Amendments of 1970 (amendments to the PHS Act of 1944) reestablish categorical grant programs to control communicable diseases such as tuberculosis, venereal disease, measles, and rubella. It also changes the name of the Communicable Disease Center to the Centers for Disease Control and broadens its concern beyond communicable diseases to other preventable conditions such as malnutrition, certain chronic health problems, and accidental injuries.

1971   The Comprehensive Health Manpower Training Act of 1971 (PHS Act amendment) includes a complex series of amendments that replace institutional grants with a new system of capitation grants in which health professions schools receive fixed sums of money for each student enrolled, contingent on increasing first-year enrollments.

The National Cancer Act is signed into law.

1972   The Social Security Amendments of 1972 make significant changes in the Medicare program to try to control growing costs.

1973   The Health Maintenance Organization Act of 1973 (amendment to the PHS Act) and amendments in 1976, 1978, and 1981 encourages the development of HMOs by specifying the basic medical services an HMO has to provide in order to be eligible for federal funding. To encourage enrollment, it mandates that every employer of 25 or more persons offer an HMO option. Later amendments mitigated the stringency of the original requirements for HMOs to be eligible for federal funding.

1974   National Health Planning and Resources Development Act of 1974 (amendment to the Public Health Services Act

PL-93-641) added two new titles, XV and XVI, to the PHS act and substantially replaced the programs established under sections 314a and 314b of the comprehensive Health Planning Act of 1966 as well as some of the provisions of the Hill-Burton Act of 1946 by creating a system of local and state planning agencies supported through federal funds.

1976   The Medical Devices Amendment of 1976 (amendment to the Federal Food, Drug, and Cosmetic Act of 1944) strengthens the regulation of medical devices, partially as a reaction to concerns over the Dalkon Shield intrauterine device.

1977   The Health Care Financing Administration (HCFA) is created to manage Medicare and Medicaid separately from the Social Security Administration.

The Health Maintenance Organization Amendments of 1977 amend the 1973 HMO Act and ease the requirements an HMO must meet to be federally qualified; qualification is required for an HMO to receive Medicare and Medicaid funds.

The Indian Health Care Improvement Act of 1977 fills gaps in the delivery of healthcare services to Native Americans, mostly through the Indian Health Service.

The Rural Health Care Services Amendments of 1977 (amendments to the Medicare and Medicaid Legislation of 1965) modifies the categories of practitioners that can provide services. Rural health clinics can be reimbursed for services provided by nurse practitioners if they meet certain requirements.

The Medicare and Medicaid Antifraud and Abuse Amendments of 1977 (amendments to the Medicare and Medicaid legislation of 1965) are passed as part of an effort to reduce fraud and abuse in the programs to help contain costs.

1980   The Omnibus Budget Reconciliation Act (OBRA) of 1980 begins a new trend of omnibus legislation covering many aspects of health and other policy areas being passed as part of the budget reconciliation process. The act is contained in the Title IX of Medicare and Medicaid Amendments of 1980.

1981   The Omnibus Budget Reconciliation Act (OBRA) of 1981 is passed. Inpatient deductible for Medicare is increased. This legislation also includes extensive changes in 46 sections, including eliminating coverage of alcohol detoxification facilities and removal of occupational therapy as a basis for entitlement for home health services.

Acquired Immune Deficiency Syndrome (AIDS) is identified.

1982   The Tax Equity and Fiscal Responsibility Act of (TEFRA) 1982 makes important changes in Medicare and Medicaid and in other health-related programs. It replaces PSROS (established by the Social Security Amendments of 1972) and eliminates requirements for local HSAs. The act also replaces PSROS with PROS and makes their use in hospitals optional for patients covered under government programs.

1983   The Social Security Amendments of 1983 include a major landmark in the Medicare program. The basic rules of the Medicare program are modified to be a prospective payment system for hospital care by basing payments to hospitals on predetermined rates per discharge for diagnosis related groups (DRGs), replacing the earlier cost-based system of reimbursement. In addition, the act authorizes a study of physician payment reform options.

1984   The Deficit Reduction Act of 1984 (DEFRA) temporarily freezes increases in physician payment under Medicare and places a specific limit on the rate of increase in DRG payment rates in the following two years. It also establishes the Medicare Participating Physician and Supplier Program (PAR), which creates two classes of physicians in regards to their relationships to the Medicare program and outlines different reimbursement depending upon whether one is classified as "participating" or "nonparticipating."

The National Organ Transplantation Act is signed into law.

The HIV virus is identified by PHS and French scientists.

1985   The Consolidated Omnibus Budget Reconciliation Act of 1985 (COBRA 1985) impacts the Medicare program by adjusting the disproportionate share payments made to hospitals that serve many poor patients.

A blood test to detect HIV is licensed.

1986   The Omnibus Budget Reconciliation Act of 1986 (OBRA 1986) alters PPS payment rate for hospitals; reduces payment amounts for capital related costs; and establishes further limits to balance billing by physicians by setting maximum allowable charges for physicians who do not participate in the PAR program.

The Omnibus Health Act of 1986 liberalizes coverage under the Medicaid program by using income up to the federal poverty line as a criterion. This change allows states to offer all pregnant women and infants up to one year coverage with a phase in schedule up to five years of age. The act also includes the National Childhood Vaccine Injury Act that establishes a federal vaccine injury compensation program system.

1987   The Omnibus Budget Reconciliation Act of 1987 (OBRA 1987) alters many aspects of both Medicare and Medicaid. For Medicare, the major changes are that the wage index used to calculate hospital payments is updated, and capital-related costs are reduced by 12 percent for fiscal year 1988 and 15 percent for fiscal year 1989. For physician payment, fees for 12 overvalued procedures are reduced, and higher fee increases are allowed for primary care than for specialized physician services. For Medicaid, states are required to cover eligible children up to age 6 with an option for up to age 8. In addition, the distinction between skilled nursing facilities and intermediate care facilities is eliminated, and provisions designed to enhance the quality of care in nursing homes are included.

1988   The National Organ Transplant Amendments of 1988 (amendments to the National Organ Transplant Act of 1984) extends the prohibition against the sale of human organs and body parts of human fetuses.

The Medicare Catastrophic Coverage Act (amendment to the Medicare act of 1965) provides the largest expansion of benefits since the creation of the program, including some added coverage for outpatient drugs and respite care.

The McKinney Act is signed into law, providing healthcare to the homeless.

1989   The Omnibus Budget Reconciliation Act of 1989 (OBRA 1989) includes provisions for minor, predominantly technical changes in the PPS such as some coverage for mental health benefits and PAP smears and small adjustments in disproportionate share rules. The major change is to begin the implementation of a resource based relative value scale (RBRVS) for physician payment, phased in over a four-year period starting with 1992. Also, a new agency, Agency for Health Care Policy and Research (AHCPR) is created to replace the National Center for Health Services Research and Technology Assessment (NCHSR). The focus of the new agency is to conduct and foster studies of healthcare quality, effectiveness and efficiency, including those on outcomes of medical care treatment.

1990   The Americans with Disabilities Act (ADA) of 1990 provides a broad range of protections for the disabled, and thus combines protections from the Civil Rights Act of 1964, the Rehabilitation Act of 1973, and the Civil Rights Restoration Act of 1988. The legislation helps the disabled toward a goal of independence and self-support.

The Ryan White Comprehensive AIDS Resources Emergency Act of 1990 (amendment to the Public Health Service Act of 1944) sets up special programs to distribute funds related to AIDS through grants.

The Omnibus Budget Reconciliation Act of 1990 (OBRA '90) includes the Patient Self-Determination Act, a variety of minor changes in PPS, and other technical adjustments to Medicare payments.

The Human Genome Project is established.

1993 The National Institutes of Health Revitalization Act of 1993 provides for some structural and budgetary changes in the operation of NIH. This act includes guidelines for the conduct of research on transplantation of human fetal tissue, and adds HIV infection to the list of excludable conditions covered by the Immigration and Nationality Act.

The Omnibus Budget Reconciliation Act of 1993 (OBRA 1993) puts into place a record five-year cut in Medicare funding and includes other changes in Medicare such as a provision to end return on equity (ROE) payments for capital to proprietary SNFs. The act reduces the rate of increase of inpatient rates for care provided in hospices, cuts laboratory fees, and freezes payments for durable medical equipment, parenteral and enteral services, and orthotics and prosthetics.

The Childhood Immunization Act supports the provision of vaccines for children eligible for Medicaid, children without health insurance, and Native American children.

The Oregon Health Plan (OHP) begins operation, after achieving a Medicaid waiver from the traditional operation of Medicaid. The Oregon Health Plan (OHP) is a public/private partnership to ensure access to healthcare for all Oregonians.

1994 The Social Security Act Amendments of 1994 make a number of technical and other changes in the Medicare program. The Maternal and Child Health block grant program is modified, as are Medicare adjusted standardized amounts for wages and wage related costs. The amendments also provide more coverage for psychologists, refine the geographic cost of practice index for physician payment, limit extra billing of physicians, and requires the creation of complete relative values for pediatric services. It also modifies durable medical equipment rules and sets in place mammography certification requirements.

The Veterans Health Programs Extension Act of 1994 adds the treatment of sexual trauma and repeals the limitation in time to seek services for this issue. The act increases research relating to women veterans and increases authority to provide priority healthcare for veterans exposed to toxic substances.

NIH-supported scientists discover the genes responsible for many cases of hereditary colon cancer, inherited breast cancer, and the most common type of kidney cancer.

1995   The Social Security Administration becomes an independent agency March 31.

1996   The Health Insurance Portability and Accountability Act of 1996 (also known as the Kennedy-Kassebaum Act, or HIPAA) improves portability and continuity of health insurance coverage in group and individual markets when an individual loses a job. It also promotes the use of medical savings accounts, improves access to long term care services and coverage and provides for changes in membership and duties of the national committee on vital and health statistics.

The Health Centers Consolidation Act of 1996 (amendment to the Public Health Service Act of 1944 and its amendments) consolidates and more clearly defines health centers, primary care services and medically underserved areas. There are special provisions for services to the homeless.

The Indian Health Care Improvement Technical Corrections Act of 1996 (amendment to the Indian Health Care Improvement Act of 1977) extends demonstration programs for direct billing of Medicare, Medicaid and other third-party payers.

The Veterans Health Care Eligibility Reform Act of 1996 amends previous veterans' healthcare legislation to reform eligibility for healthcare provided by the Department of Veterans' Affairs. The act also makes changes related to the provision of care in the extent and amount provided in advance by authorization legislation. More care is provided for women veterans, including readjustment counseling and mental healthcare. Special studies on hospice care begin.

The Ryan White Care Act Amendments of 1996 (amendments to the Ryan White Comprehensive AIDS Resources

Emergency Act of 1990) sets new definitions of eligible areas and eligible population numbers, and makes modifications in membership of the councils to aid in distribution of funds.

Welfare reform is enacted under the Personal Responsibility and Work Opportunity Reconciliation Act.

The Health Insurance Portability and Accountability Act of 1996 (HIPAA) establishes the Medicare Integrity Program, which provides funds for program integrity activities.

1997   The State Children's Health Insurance Program is established.

The Balanced Budget Act of 1997 (BBA) includes a wide range of changes in provider payments to slow growth in Medicare spending as part of legislation to balance the federal budget. In a large new effort, the Medicare+Choice program, a new structure for Medicare HMOs and other private health plans, is offered to beneficiaries.

1998   The Initiative to Eliminate Racial and Ethnic Disparities in Health begins.

As a way to improve the access of the general public to information about Medicare, the internet site www.Medicare.gov is launched to provide updated information.

1999   The Ticket to Work and Work Incentives Improvement Act of 1999 is signed, making it possible for millions of Americans with disabilities to join the workforce without fear of losing their Medicaid and Medicare coverage. It also modernizes the employment services system for people with disabilities.

An initiative on combating bioterrorism is launched.

2000   Human genome sequencing is published.

The Medicare, Medicaid, and SCHIP Benefits Improvement and Protection Act (BIPA) of 2000 continues to modify payments to providers, and increases Medicare payments to providers and Medicare+Choice plans.

2001   The Centers for Medicare & Medicaid Services is created, replacing the Health Care Financing Administration.

2002   The Public Health Security and Bioterrorism Preparedness and Response Act of 2002 is signed; it includes a number of public health measures.

2003   The Consolidated Appropriations Resolution (CAR) of 2003 increases payments for Medicare for some hospitals, updates the physician fee schedule, and makes some changes in premium payments for some Part B recipients.

The Medicare Prescription Drug, Improvement, and Modernization Act of 2003 (MMA) is passed by the House (220–215) and the Senate (54–44) in November and signed into law (Public Law 108-173) by President Bush. This provides a new outpatient prescription drug benefit under Medicare beginning in 2006.

2004   A temporary Medicare-approved drug discount card program begins.

2005   Medicare begins covering "Welcome to Medicare" physicals, along with other preventive services, such as cardiovascular screening, blood tests, and diabetes screening tests. Medicare also begins education and outreach activities to implement the 2006 prescription drug benefit. The first open enrollment period for the new Part D drug benefit, in which Medicare beneficiaries can enroll in a Medicare Prescription Drug Plan (PDP) or a Medicare Advantage Prescription Drug Plan (MAPD) begins.

2006   The Medicare Drug Benefit begins.

The State of Massachusetts passes the Massachusetts Health Care Plan, now better known as Mass Health.

2007   Medicare beneficiaries with higher incomes (greater than $80,000/individual; $160,000/couple) begin to pay a higher monthly Part B premium.

The Medicare, Medicaid, and SCHIP Extension Act of 2007 (PL110–173) is signed into law. The act prevents a 10.1 percent reduction in Medicare physician payments that had been scheduled for 2008 and gives physicians a 0.5 percent increase through June 30, 2008.

2008 The Medicare Improvements for Patients and Providers Act of 2008 (MIPPA) is signed into law (PL 110-275). The bill prevents a reduction in physician fees through the end of 2008, and increases fees by 1.1 percent through 2009. Because these changes are supposed to be revenue neutral, the cost of the postponement of physician fee cuts is offset by cutting bonus payments to Medicare Advantage plans.

Medicare beneficiaries with incomes exceeding $82,000/individual and $164,000/couple pay income-related Part B premiums of up to $238.40.

The Paul Wellstone and Pete Domenici Mental Health Parity and Addiction Equity Act of 2008 is passed as part of the stimulus package. The law ends discrimination against consumers of mental health and substance abuse treatment services in many health insurance plans.

2009–2010 The US House of Representatives passes the Senate bill to reform healthcare in March, 2010 by a vote of 220–211. The House also passes a bill which then goes back to the Senate to modify some versions of the Senate bill. The original Senate version was passed in late 2009. The modification bill (known as the reconciliation bill) passes 56–43, and then is approved by the House by a vote of 22 to 207, and signed by President Obama. The bill is now known as the Affordable Care Act (ACA). The overall bill was signed by President Obama on March 23, 2010.

2011 Under the ACA, insurance companies are required to spend 80 to 85 percent of premiums on medical care, provide free preventive care under Medicare, and half-priced brand-name prescription drugs as a way to reduce the Medicare donut hole.

2012 ACA allows physicians incentives to join together and form accountable care organizations in which doctors coordinate patient care, improve quality, and reduce unnecessary hospital admissions; health programs must report racial, ethnic, and language data about insured people to help reduce health disparities.

2013   Additional funding to Medicaid provides for programs that choose to cover preventive services for people; states must pay primary care providers at least at the Medicare rate. States will receive additional funding for children not eligible for Medicaid as part of CHI; a pilot program of bundling payments by episodes of care with a flat fee begins.

2014   States have certified exchanges and begin enrollment in fall of 2013 with care beginning in 2014. People are required to purchase basic health insurance coverage. Medicaid expands in states that agree to participate. Companies may no longer refuse to sell or renew coverage due to preexisting conditions and from charging more due to gender or health status.

Changes Due to Take Place in the Future as Part of ACA Legislation

2015   Increase federal match by 23 percentage points in the Children's Health Insurance Program (CHIP) match rate up to a cap of 100 percent, starting in October 2015.

2016   Healthcare choice compacts will be permitted by states to allow insurers to sell policies in any state participating in the compact, beginning in October 2016.

2018   ACA will impose an excise tax on insurers of employer-sponsored health plans with aggregate expenses that exceed $10,200 for individual coverage and $27,500 for family coverage.

Access to care Ability of persons needing healthcare services to obtain appropriate care in a timely manner. While access to care is not the same as having health insurance coverage, having health insurance coverage, either private or public such as Medicare or Medicaid, is a major factor in having access to care.

Acute care Short-term care, often of an intense nature and often for injury or illness. This type of care can include hospitalization, just for a short-term, intense problem rather than a long-term, chronic problem.

Affordable Care Act (ACA) Act passed in the Obama administration in 2010 to increase healthcare insurance coverage in the United States. Certain provisions begin at different points in time, with the major beginning of healthcare exchanges for people to buy insurance through this act in 2014. The act ends preexisting condition exclusions for children and allows young adults under age 26 to remain on parents' insurance. Lifetime limits on most benefits are banned for new health insurance plans, and companies must publicly justify unreasonable rate hikes. Preventive health services must be covered without copayments.

AHRQ Agency for Health Care Research and Quality (formerly AHCPR); deals with issues of healthcare policy, health services research, health quality issues; and health practice guidelines. Also conducts several important surveys to obtain data on healthcare expenditures and some hospital-related data.

An earlier version of the agency before AHRQ and AHCPR was NCHSR, National Center for Health Services Research.

Ambulatory care   Sometimes also called outpatient care. This is care given to people in a doctor's office, outpatient center, or other special parts of hospitals, for which patients do not need to stay overnight in any type of formal healthcare facility.

Assisted living facilities   These are places where people live as they age and have some type of help provided. Some places are really independent living options where people have their own apartments, with the assistance being the availability of transportation to shopping and to healthcare facilities, and the presence within the overall facility of dining facilities, often with one or two meals a day included as part of the basic rental fee. Sometimes, much smaller personal living places are included, in an assisted living wing in which there may be a small bedroom, bathroom, and a living room that combines a sitting and eating area with limited kitchen facilities and daily supervision of a person's medication. People often have three meals a day in these settings. In most states, there is very limited regulation of these types of long-term care options, as contrasted with nursing home settings.

Capitation   A set amount or a flat rate that is paid to cover a person's medical care for a specified period of time, often a month or a year.

CDC   Centers for Disease Control and Prevention, the federal agency that includes the National Center for Health Statistics (NCHS) and has responsibility for a variety of prevention-oriented programs, including chronic diseases as well as acute problems and infectious disease. It is the major federal health agency that deals with epidemiology and disease control, especially outbreaks of infectious diseases such as seasonal flu or the H1NI flu concern of the winter of 2009–2010 or the recent concern over the Ebola virus in other countries.

Chronic disease   Medical conditions that persist over time. Chronic problems may lead to permanent healthcare problems. Examples of chronic diseases include diabetes, heart disease, and chronic obstructive pulmonary disease. Chronic care can occur in many settings, such as outpatient, hospitals, or long-term care facilities.

CMS   Center for Medicare and Medicaid Services. Formerly, this agency was known as HCFA, the Health Care Financing Administration. This is the agency that administers the Medicare, Medicaid, and SCHIP programs.

Copayment   A portion of healthcare expenses that the patient must provide. Generally, a health insurance plan or HMO will specify this to the insured person. A copayment is generally paid each time a person receives healthcare services.

Deductible   A portion of healthcare costs that the insured person must pay first before insurance payments begin. Generally, most plans provide a coverage year, which could coincide with the calendar year, or a different time frame such as from July through June. A person will pay the costs for healthcare that they receive until this amount is met and then generally, health insurance will begin to cover the costs, often along with a copayment.

DHHS   Department of Health and Human Services. The overall federal agency that deals with many health-related issues. Agencies such as the National Institutes of Health are part of this agency.

Disability   Physical or mental handicap that results from injury or illness. These often impact a person's ability to perform a variety of life tasks. For example, a person who is blind has a visual disability, and a person who is deaf has a hearing disability. Examples of other types of physical disabilities are the need to use a wheelchair or a prosthetic device for movement of the legs and ambulation or for movement of the hands in the upper body.

DRG   Diagnosis-related group. This is the current payment approach used for Medicare hospital payments. Rather than paying for specific services as they occur in the hospital, hospital charges are paid for a bundled group of all services as related to a federally specified list of diagnoses. This approach of paying for hospital care has also been incorporated by some private health insurance companies.

Entitlement programs   Healthcare programs that certain categories of people are entitled to, such as most people at age 65 being entitled to Medicare because they paid payroll taxes during their employed years.

Fee-for-service   Payment of specific fees (generally to a physician) for each service that a patient receives, such as an office examination, a shot (immunization), or a diagnostic test.

Formulary   List of acceptable prescription drugs that a health plan or managed care company allows. In many health coverages, there may be higher copayments for nongeneric formulary drugs than for generic versions of formulary drugs. If a drug is not listed in the formulary of the health insurance plan (including Medicare drug coverage plans), then no payment will be made for that prescription.

Gatekeeper physician   Generally, a primary care physician who functions as the regular source of care for a patient and who must approve the use of specialists and other services, most often as part of a managed care plan.

GDP   Gross domestic product. It is a measure of all the goods and services produced by a nation in a given year.

Generalist   A family practice, general internal medicine, or general pediatrics physician. These types of physicians often function as gatekeepers within certain managed care systems.

HMO   Health maintenance organization. A type of managed care organization that generally provides comprehensive medical care for a set predetermined annual fee per employee, generally with only modest copayments and small or no deductibles, although there have been some trends of increases in sizes of copayments to keep basic health insurance costs lower.

Home health services Nursing, special therapy services such as physical therapy, and health-related homemaker services that are provided to patients in their home, generally because the patients have a chronic illness or a disability that makes the patient unable to leave home to receive services.

Hospice services An array of special services for patients who are dying. Generally, these are a blend of medical, spiritual, legal, and family support services that can be delivered in the patient's home, a nursing home, or a special facility designed for this purpose.

Hospital services The healthcare services patients receive while spending the night in a hospital. Similar to inpatient services.

Independent practice association (IPA) Legal entity that physicians in private practice join so that the organization can represent them in the negotiation of contracts with managed care organizations.

Infant mortality rate Deaths that occur to infants in the first year of life. This is usually considered one of the best indicators of how well a country's healthcare system is working.

Infectious diseases Diseases that are transmitted in various ways, through the air, through water, and sexually. Currently, many of the most important infectious diseases are transmitted sexually and through the blood stream, such as HIV.

Inpatient services Services received while a patient is in a hospital or nursing home, while staying overnight.

Insurance carrier The insurer.

Insured The person who contracts with an insurance company for coverage; also known as the policy holder or the subscriber.

Lifecare communities Places where, in exchange for a one-time entrance fee plus a monthly maintenance fee, a person receives a guarantee of assisted living, personal care, and nursing home services as needed.

Lifetime cap   Maximum amount of money a health insurance policy will pay over the lifetime of the insured person. Limitations on these caps have been major issues for people who develop serious health problems. The ACA does not allow such caps in health insurance plans.

Long-term care   Services received as part of extended care needed for people with chronic illnesses, mental illnesses, or serious disabilities. These services are often provided in nursing homes but can also be provided as part of home-based services or assisted living services and often focus on basic daily needs.

Managed care   A system of provision and payment for health-care that unites the functions of health insurance and the actual delivery of care.

MCO   Managed care organization.

Medicaid   A joint federal-state program that provides health insurance coverage to many poor people in the United States.

Medicare   The federal program that provides health insurance coverage to older adults and to some people with disabilities. Part A covers hospital costs, Part B covers physician and provider costs, and Part D is a newer drug coverage option. The major payer for health insurance for most people over age 65 in the United States, although many people also have supplemental health insurance coverage (sometimes called Medigap plans) that pays for things not covered or not covered completely by Medicare in addition to a Part D drug plan.

Medigap   Commercial health insurance policies purchased by people with Medicare coverage to cover expenses not covered by Medicare; the insurance also provides coverage for certain other costs within Medicare, such as required copayments and deductibles for certain services.

Morbidity   Sickness.

Mortality   Death.

Neonatal death rates   Refers to deaths of infants in the first 28 days of life, generally considered more sensitive to genetic factors and conditions during birth, as contrasted to the infant mortality rate.

NIH   National Institutes of Health. This is the major research arm of the federal government, as related to health. It includes institutes such as the National Cancer Institute, and its headquarters are located in Bethesda, Maryland. It is the major federal funder of health research and also conducts some of its own research.

Nursing homes   Facilities where the most seriously ill older adults (and some younger people) with chronic health problems receive long-term care. These types of institutions are subject to federal and state regulation, and generally have some registered nurses available at all times (in contrast to assisted living facilities).

Organized medicine   Refers to the activities of physicians, generally to protect their own interests, such as through groups such as the American Medical Association.

Outcome   Result of healthcare delivery; of great interest now as a way to measure the effectiveness of the healthcare delivery system.

Out of pocket costs   Costs of healthcare that are paid by the patient, the consumer of services; depending on the type of health insurance a person has, this would include required deductibles and copayments for care.

Outpatient services   Provided healthcare services that are not part of an overnight stay in a hospital (as contrasted to inpatient services).

Payer   Party that actually makes the payment for services covered by an insurance policy. Generally, the payer is the same as the insurer.

Physician-hospital organization   A legal entity that is formed between a hospital and a physician group, generally to share a market, patients, and other mutual interests.

Preexisting condition   Condition (either physical or mental) that existed prior to the beginning of an insurance policy. Some policies exclude these kinds of conditions. Generally, workplace policies will not. Removal of these conditions has been a major topic of recent healthcare reform discussions.

Preferred provider organization (PPO)   These types of organizations are related to managed care plans. Often, insurance companies make a contractual arrangement with a group of providers or individual providers for provision of services, typically at a discounted fee.

Premiums   Amount charged by an insurance company for a policy.

Primary care   Medical care provided in an office or clinic setting by a provider such as a doctor, physician's assistant, or nurse practitioner. Generally, this is the first level of patient contact within the healthcare delivery system and the entry point into healthcare.

Prospective payment system (PPS)   In this type of payment system, how much is to be paid for a particular service is predetermined, as contrasted with retrospective reimbursement. The DRG payment system for hospital care under Medicare is an example of a prospective payment system.

RBRVS (resource-based relative value system)   A system in place within Medicare to determine physician fees. Each treatment or visit with a physician is assigned a "relative value" based on the training, skill, and time that is required to treat the condition.

Reimbursement   Amount paid to a provider (e.g., doctor, hospital) by the insurance company or managed care group. This payment may be only a portion of what the provider charges. In a managed care setting, the amount may have been negotiated in advance.

Retrospective reimbursement   The amount to be paid is determined on the basis of the actual costs incurred, generally after services have been delivered.

Safety net   Programs that enable people to receive healthcare services (as well as many other social services) even if they lack personal resources to pay for those services. Medicaid is an example of a safety-net program in healthcare, as are community health centers. These are generally government programs.

SCHIP   State Child Health Insurance Program. This program was passed in 1997 as part of the Balanced Budget Act of that year. At the time, it was the largest expansion of health coverage since Medicare and Medicaid. It is a joint federal-state healthcare program and allows states to provide health insurance coverage for children of the working poor.

Single-payer   a proposal for healthcare reform that emphasizes the creation of a single organization, typically a government agency, to pay all healthcare claims. While many experts argue this is the best and least expensive way to provide healthcare access to a population, it has not been a popular approach in recent rounds of discussion of U.S. healthcare reform.

UCR (usual, customary, and reasonable)   Maximum charges that an insurer will reimburse for a specific service. Typically, each insurance company determines what its own UCR is, as part of community or statewide surveys of what providers charge.

Uncompensated care   Services provided to consumers as charity without the person paying for the services.

Welfare programs   Means-tested programs that provide services, whether health or social, to those with low incomes. In healthcare, Medicaid is an example of a welfare program.

About the Authors

Jennie Jacobs Kronenfeld is a professor in the Sociology Program in the Sanford School of Social and Family Dynamics, Arizona State University. Her research areas are medical sociology along with aging and the life course, with a special focus on health policy, healthcare utilization, and health behavior. She serves as the editor of the research annual *Research in the Sociology of Health Care,* published each year by Emerald Press. She is coeditor of *Health* and associate editor in chief of the *American Journal of Health Promotion.*

Michael Kronenfeld, MLS, MBA, AHIP, is the University Librarian and head of the A. T. Still Memorial Library at the A. T. Still University of the Health Sciences. He has spent most of his 40-year career as a medical librarian in a number of settings, including a school of public health, a county teaching hospital in a major urban area, and the last 12 years in a health sciences university. In addition to coauthoring the two editions of this book, he has also published over 25 articles in peer-reviewed journals and been active in professional organizations, including the Medical Library Association, where he has received several national awards, including the Ida and George Eliot Prize in 2001, which is presented annually for a work published in the preceding calendar year that has been judged most effective in furthering medical librarianship.